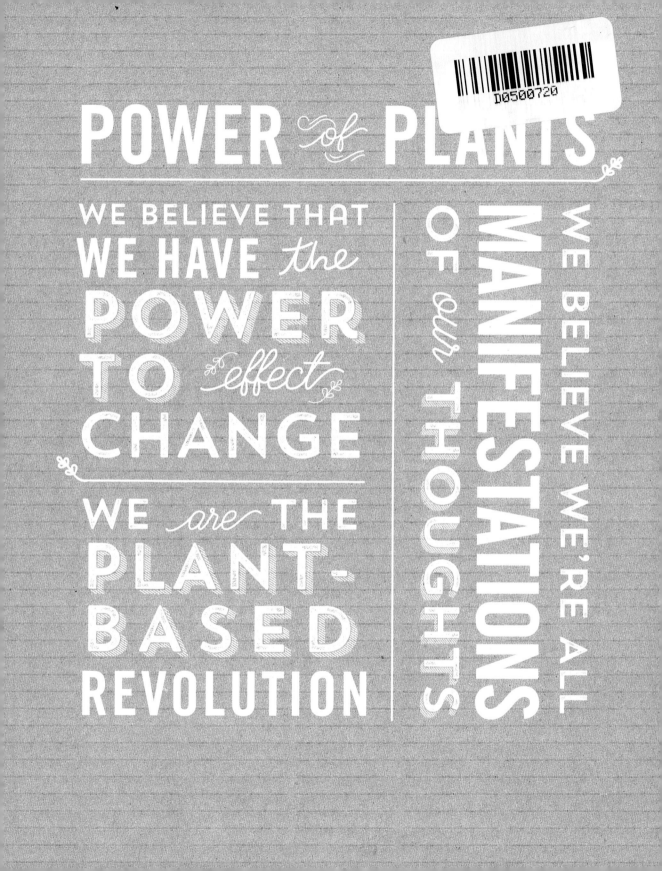

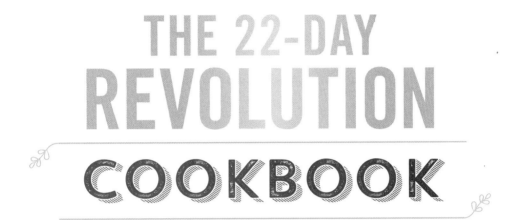

THE 22-DAY
REVOLUTION
COOKBOOK

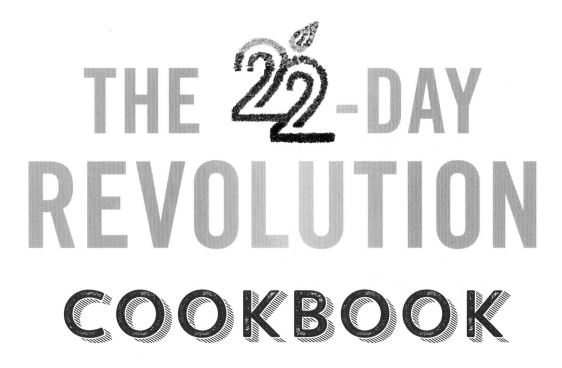

THE 22-DAY REVOLUTION COOKBOOK

Unleash the Life-Changing Health Benefits

of a Plant-Based Diet

MARCO BORGES

CELEBRA
New York

CELEBRA
Published by Berkley
An imprint of Penguin Random House LLC
375 Hudson Street, New York, New York 10014

Photos courtesy of Ben Coppelman

Library of Congress Cataloging-in-Publication Data
Names: Borges, Marco.
Title: The 22-day revolution cookbook: Unleash the life-changing health benefits of a plant-based diet/ Marco Borges.
Other titles: Twenty-two day revolution cookbook | Twenty two day revolution cookbook
Description: New York, New York : Celebra, 2016. | "A Celebra book."
Identifiers: LCCN 2016012530 (print) | LCCN 2016021499 (ebook) | ISBN 9781101989586 (hardback) | ISBN 9781101989609 (ebook)
Subjects: LCSH: Vegetarianism. | Diet. | BISAC: COOKING/General. | COOKING/Health & Healing / Weight Control. | HEALTH & FITNESS/Diets. | LCGFT: Cookbooks.
Classification: LCC TX392 .B636 2016 (print) | LCC TX392 (ebook) | DDC 641.5/636—dc23
LC record available at https://lccn.loc.gov/2016012530

First Edition: September 2016

Printed in the United States of America
1   3   5   7   9   10   8   6   4   2

Jacket photography and styling by Ben Coppelman
Interior photography by Ben Coppelman
Interior photography styling by Elizabeth Reinhardt and Ben Coppelman
Jacket design by Emily Osborne
Book design by Pauline Neuwirth

To Mila, Maximo, Mateo, Marco Jr., and Marilyn

I love you with all of my heart.

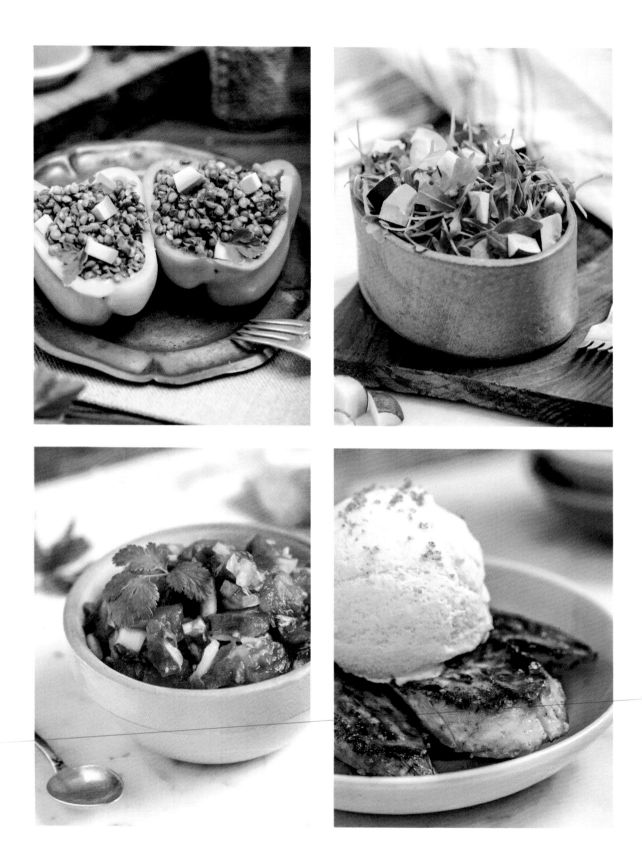

CONTENTS

FOREWORD

BY RYAN SEACREST

WHEN I WAS A KID, one of my favorite foods was nachos.

Nachos, pizza, chips, candy—like many other growing boys, I really loved junk food. The problem is that the "junk food" didn't love me back. I became overweight, and I didn't feel great about myself. I was self-conscious and wary of social situations like pool parties. In fact, I insisted on wearing my Bon Jovi T-shirt *in* the pool.

In high school, I started working out and eating healthier, and I overcame many of my insecurities, as my body became more of what I wanted it to be. Honestly, though, I struggled with my weight for a long time. Part of it was that I just love food. (Who doesn't?) The other part, maybe the more important part, was that I really didn't understand the true science of food and how it applied to my body, mind, and soul.

I met Marco Borges about five years ago. I had heard great things about how he helped people learn to lead healthier lives and achieve what they once thought impossible. What struck me most when I first met him was just how thoughtfully he approached talking about my health. He shared with me that the connectivity between food and fitness was paramount, but he also was focused on full-body health, which meant not only eating a balanced diet of whole foods but also developing fitness programs that worked for me and my lifestyle.

With Marco's guidance, I tried the 22-Day Revolution program and ate a vegan, plant-based diet for the first time. He's a terrific teacher who is patient, knowledgeable, and realistic. He broke down the common mistakes, barriers, and misconceptions about eating plant based, and I learned how to build lean muscle mass without eating meat and processed protein supplements. I was surprised by how easily I was able to adapt to eating plant-based, and soon it became second nature to choose a vegan option at a restaurant or to reach for veggies and hummus for a quick snack.

And most important, I saw firsthand how a plant-based diet can and will change your life—not just your waistline but also your brain. Within the first week of beginning the program, I felt energized in a way that, given my long days and busy schedule, is very tough to achieve and maintain. I felt mentally sharper and quicker. And most of all, I felt strong and powerful physically. That feeling was a far cry from the overweight boy hiding at the community pool. Now, whether I'm on the red carpet, out with friends, or at the gym, I am more confident, happier, and healthier than ever before.

The 22-Day Revolution Cookbook is an incredible tool, as you can tailor the book's 150 recipes to your individual goals. It also helps you navigate how to maintain this program even when you are eating out at restaurants, which is always a challenge for many of us.

This book isn't about converting people into being vegan. It's about teaching people to incorporate more plant-based foods into their life and creating long-term healthy habits, by eating exclusively plant-based over the course of 22 days. The degree to which anyone choses to eat plant-based after a 22-day cycle will be equal to the degree to which they benefit. The goal is to help readers live their best lives and be the best version of themselves.

Marco has certainly set me on a course to be my best self, and, sadly, that means no more nachos—although they remain my go-to on cheat days! Living by the 22 Day mandates also means that I get to enjoy these delicious and healthful recipes, which make me feel my absolute best. I say that's a pretty great trade-off.

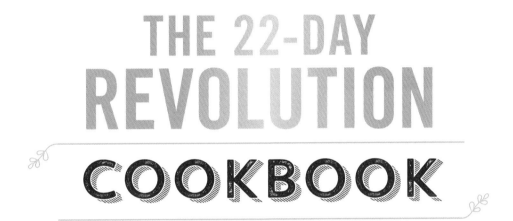

THE 22-DAY
REVOLUTION
COOKBOOK

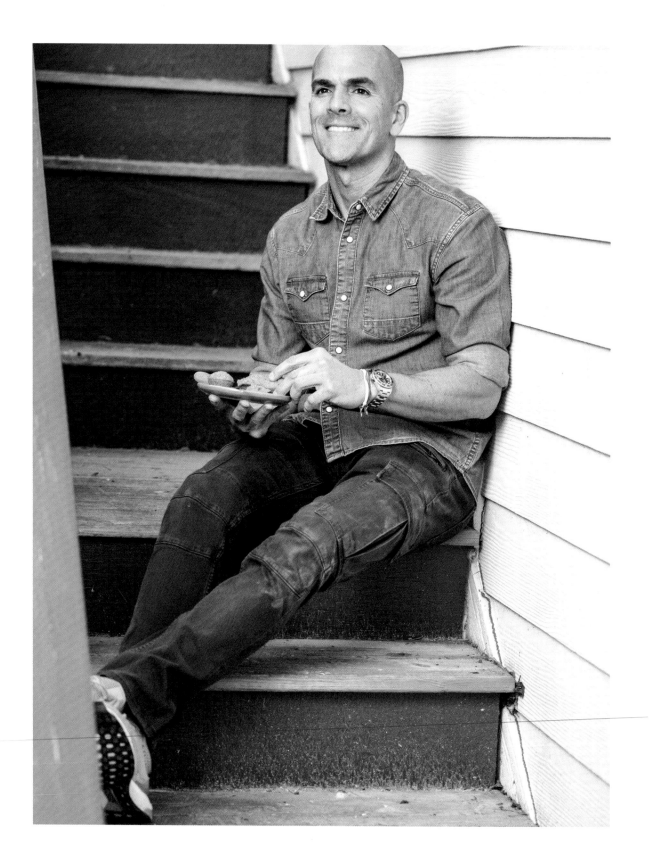

INTRODUCTION

*The health of nations is more important
than the wealth of nations.*

—WILL DURANT

WELCOME TO THE 22-DAY FAMILY

If you are holding this book, you're already a part of our 22-Day family. In my world, a family is a place where you feel safe, where you can be vulnerable, and where you can find the strength to make positive changes. Together, we support one another in achieving goals, in learning more, in getting up and trying our best even when it doesn't come easy.

My goal in writing this book is to help you bring optimum wellness home with you by arming you with tools for success.

Some people go to spas to lose weight. They're making it easier for themselves, which is something we should all be doing. But what happens on the following Monday when they get home and there's nothing in the kitchen but sugary snacks loaded with extra salt and unhealthy fats? Boom, there go all those good intentions.

A spa is a wonderful reset. But by outsourcing your environment, by letting someone else shop for ingredients and prepare your meals, by having meals portioned by somebody else, you are missing out on learning how to take care of yourself by yourself. That makes it that much more challenging to stick to the new routines you've been introduced to, no matter how well-meaning and well-intentioned you are, no matter how committed you are to the idea of increasing your well-being.

I wrote this book, and all of my books, because health that begins at home is sustainable. It can last. When you learn to prepare plant-based meals for yourself, without relying on a chef, you are taking a closer look at what your nutrition consists of. When you know how to cook healthful foods, when you understand the importance of nutrition to your health, you have the tools to make healthy choices wherever you are, even at a friend's Fourth of July barbecue or yearly winter holiday bash. When you learn simple exercise routines that you can do at home, you never have to worry about the weather or the car or the traffic getting in the way of your fitness.

That's why in my own home, I have raised my children with consciousness about health. In my household, nutrition is common conversation. They hear plenty about our food and how important it is to our well-being, and exercising and how important that is for our well-being. And they don't just hear about it. They live it. We all play sports and regularly spend time outdoors running around being silly. We take family trips to the market and to local farms. My children can spot organic produce from a distance and they are always the first to leap for it. A family treat is organic fruit cups and organic roasted summer squash. My wife is as passionate as I am about healthful living and healthful eating, and I have learned so much from her about different foods and cooking over the course of our relationship. Some of my favorites that she makes are her Carrot Walnut Mini Muffins and Lentil Tabbouleh and, yes, you will find those recipes in this book.

Why am I so proud of all of this? Because in teaching my children about these things, I am giving them the gift of health.

In our family, food and love come wrapped together, as it does in all families. But that food has all of the colors of the rainbow, and it grows in gardens and is not processed into shapes with added colors in a processing plant. Plants, not processing plants. Whole foods for our whole family—and the whole life goodness that plants give us.

JOIN THE REVOLUTION

The 22-Day Revolution is about upending the way you eat, resetting your habits, and checking the old way of doing things at the door. It's about walking into a new life in which you feel energetic and vibrant and in which you're taking care of your health and losing excess weight. The revolution is about eating real foods. Fresh foods. Whole foods. Plant-based foods. Foods that are full of vitamins, full of minerals, full of proteins and carbohydrates and the healthy fats that keep all of your body's systems running smoothly—and let you live your life to the max.

I've seen it happen so many times with my clients and with people I love (and sometimes these wind up being the very same people). Men and women of all ages come to me because they are sluggish or out of sorts or because they want to lose five pounds or ten or fifty—and I introduce them to plants, and their lives change. Their thoughts sharpen. Their bodies strengthen.

That's the result of the kind of eating you'll be learning about in this book. And that's why I wrote this book—to give those of you who are new to plant-based eating a whole bunch of recipes to check out, and to give those of you who have already joined the revolution and seen all the benefits some fresh new choices at meal-times.

Whether you've tried 22 Days before or you're new to the program, this book can be used however you need it:

- If you're curious about plant-based meals and you want to try some delicious new recipes that burst with flavor as well as vitamins
- If you want to lose five, ten or even fifty pounds and you've been longing for a doable diet program that works
- If you don't like the rigidity of some menu plans, but you appreciate planned menus
- If you need a reset or your habits need a check-in, whether you've been indulging over the holidays, you've been celebrating too much and too often, or you've got an event coming up that you want to feel and look your best for
- If you want to transition from counting calories to understanding what it means to truly feel full
- If you've got a lot of weight to lose and you want a comprehensive eating program and diet that offers a fast, doable way to lose weight and improve your health
- If you're suffering from chronic illnesses caused by overeating and eating overly processed foods and meats and poultries that are full of antibiotics and hormones, not to mention artificial flavors and colors
- If you're already at your dream weight and you want to stay there and get off the seesaw of weight gain and loss
- If you're an athlete who wants to use plant-based eating to give you a competitive advantage

Whoever you are, whatever you need, this book is for you. Because this book is a cookbook and so much more. It's also a flexible guide to eating. It's a teaching tool to wake up your taste buds and wake up your consciousness. It's a weight-loss guide. It's a flexible system that you can customize fully, day by day, to get the most out of your life while you begin to eat the foods that make you feel more amazing day after day.

Whether you are new to the program or you have already accomplished your very own 22-Day Revolution, you'll be able to use this book to create your own program, personalize it based on your goals and your eating habits, and discover some new recipes made with delicious, life-giving PLANTS.

MY OWN JOURNEY TO EATING PLANTS

When people ask me how long I have been eating plants, I have a ready answer: about ten years. But the truth is that my journey to eating plants has taken me all of my life, when I really think about it. In my family, we didn't generally eat plant-based foods. We ate heavily processed and, quite often, fried foods. In my family, when I was growing up, food was also love, but it wasn't necessarily HEALTH. I take great pride in the fact that our boys and daughter are growing up with all the advantages of a plant-based diet, which are so many and which we will talk about over the course of this book.

As a kid, I discovered fitness and working out because of an uncle who was very much into fitness, and my career as an exercise physiologist came out of those early lessons about weights and how I could change and improve my body with some sweat and effort. Fitness has always been a part of my relationship with health, and you will get the most out of this book if you are balancing your plant-based eating with some good old-fashioned exercise. But the key to health is in your food. On your plate and at the end of your fork.

My food aha moment came to me when eating pastries for breakfast led to a rash. A discussion about allergies with the school nurse tipped me off to the fact that food can affect how we feel. Thinking about that and learning more about how what we eat affects our health—especially as I trained more, built up my body—taught me that the way I ate mattered. I learned about eating carbohydrates for energy and protein to build muscles. I learned about healthy fats and how good those are for my body and my brain.

And I learned about plants. About the high quality of nutrition available to us in plants. All plants. Seeds. Nuts. Legumes. Grains. Green vegetables. Stone fruit. Berries. My journey to plant-based eating took years. I've been plant-based for a decade, and I've never felt better. But I didn't just flip a switch. I took some time, I learned, I paid attention, and I saw how I felt when I stopped eating processed foods, stopped eating dairy, stopped eating meat, chicken, and eggs. I ate fish for a while, but then I stopped. Now I eat completely plant-based, and whenever possible, I teach my family, friends, and clients about eating plant-based as well.

And we all—my family, my clients, and I—reap the benefits because a plant-based diet is the foundation of optimum wellness.

WHAT IS PLANT-BASED?

I love plant-based foods. So do my clients. That's why this program works. That's what makes it so sustainable, why you can eat like this for years and just keep reaping the benefits. Because it is the way that nature intended you to eat. With 22 Days, there are no tricks. There are just a lot of treats. Treats that taste good—and are good for you. That's the foundation of the foods you'll be introduced to with 22 Days.

You'll see the word "vegan" in this book, and you'll read a lot about plant-based foods. Why not just say vegan all of the time? I mean, 22 Days is vegan, right? Yup, it's vegan, but it's more than vegan. It's not about what we're leaving out. It's about what we're putting in.

Vegan means that you don't eat meat, don't eat poultry or fish or dairy. That means that candy bars that leave out the animal products are vegan, which means that you can eat only vegan candy bars, be a vegan, and still be completely overweight and unhealthy.

But I don't want you to be overweight! I don't want you to be unhealthy! I want you to reach your desired weight. I want you to be healthy. That's why I'm teaching you about plant-based eating. Because it's not just about leaving out the milk, leaving out the eggs, leaving out the fish and poultry and meat. It's about putting in the carrots. Putting in the sesame seeds, the quinoa, the black beans and the salsa and the freshest, crispiest bright green salads and the creamiest, most amazing puddings and the spiciest, most satisfying pastas. It's about putting in the plants—whole plants, nutrition-rich plants, life-giving plants.

The 22-Day Revolution Cookbook is perfect for vegans and vegetarians because it is vegan! But it's also so much more. I've said it before and I'll say it again: When we say plant-based, we mean plants, not food made in a plant.

PLANT PROTEIN: Many plants have protein, not just the obvious sources. Yes, lentils and rice are beautiful sources of complete protein. But you can also get protein from broccoli. Yes, broccoli. As well as from peas, mushrooms, spinach . . .

NUTS AND SEEDS: Almond butter on your crackers, sunflower seeds in your salads, chia seeds in your pudding . . . nuts and seeds are bountiful sources of fats and of proteins. So pack them in lunch boxes, add them to recipes. Almond milk is dreamy and wonderful to drink. Sesame seeds are the basis of our creamy Tahini Dressing. Chia seeds are a brilliant source of energy and vitality, and so are flaxseeds and pumpkin seeds. . . .

GREEN VEGGIES: The grass is always greener, but the kale is even greener. This is where all the good stuff is. Vitamins, minerals, and fiber—and green veggies also come dressed up in purple and orange and yellow, as a trip to the farmers' market in the summertime will show (check out the rainbow chard). As well as the requisite kale and spinach, check out chard, watercress, and arugula. . . .

FRUITS: This is where the rainbow lives. You've got your basic apples and pears and bananas, your seasonal peaches and apricots, your tropical mangoes and pineapples . . . and don't forget those bright red and blue and purple berries. . . .

VEGGIES: The other side of the rainbow. The more colors on your plate, the better. Red beets, orange and yellow peppers, green zucchini, indigo and violet eggplants . . .

HEALTHY STARCHES: Whole grains and root vegetables offer carbohydrates that are complex and packed with nutrition and energy. Sweet potatoes in orange and purple; whole grain rice in black and brown and purple; quinoa, which offers plenty of protein along with those yummy carbs . . . and don't forget the steel-cut oats, a warming winter breakfast staple.

With 22 Days, if you need to lose weight, you'll lose weight. You'll remind yourself what it feels like to feel full. And you will wake your senses up, reminding yourself how good healthy can taste. And how good healthy can feel.

Every day, you'll have more abundant energy. You'll have fewer regrets or moments of guilt.

Every week, you'll see the weight come off. You'll feel more revitalized and aware.

In 22 Days, you'll feel better than you have in ages, and you'll want to keep enjoying the best of your life.

> **VEGETARIAN:** Skips meat, poultry, and fish. Goes for dairy and eggs, grains, and vegetables.
>
> **VEGAN:** Skips meat, poultry, fish, milk, eggs, and honey (anything that comes from an animal). Goes for grains, vegetables, and fruit and may choose processed vegan foods.
>
> **PLANT-BASED:** Skips meat, poultry, fish, milk, eggs (anything that comes from an animal), and processed foods. Eats 100 percent plants: grains, legumes, beans, vegetables, fruit, seeds, and nuts.

THE CONNECTION BETWEEN PLANTS AND HEALTH

What we eat, what we feed ourselves, what we feed our families—this is the basis of how we walk around feeling all the time. Do you feel well physically? Do you feel well emotionally? Do you feel well mentally?

There are some symptoms of modern life that too many people have begun to take for granted, as if it is really natural or normal to experience:

- fatigue and exhaustion
- stomachaches after meals
- the feeling that you wish you "hadn't eaten that"
- heartburn and indigestion
- a bloated belly
- weight gain
- weight fluctuation
- obesity
- chronic illnesses like type 2 diabetes
- headaches
- trouble sleeping
- poor skin

If any of this sounds familiar to you, it's possible that your food is to blame. If it comes in a plastic wrapper, can be found in the freezer section, or can be microwaved to be ready in under a minute, it may not really be food, and it is probably why you feel weighed down, why you feel tired, and why you feel sick.

Are you ready for food that makes you healthier? Are you ready for meals that make you stronger? How about trimmer, fitter, healthier, and happier? The recipes in this book, the menus, and the programs are designed to lead you toward health. Food and health go hand in hand. Quit the meat, the dairy, and the eggs. Choose the fruits, the vegetables, and the grains. And you will see how quickly good health follows.

The fact is that plants keep our bodies in their best possible condition. They help us avoid the preventable diseases that have become a plague in our society. Studies show that eating red meat and processed meat increases risks of cancer and cardio-vascular disease.[*] Meanwhile, researchers have found that eating plants reduces cardiovascular disease.[†] Heart attacks are a major killer of men and women. Doesn't it make sense for us to embrace an eating style that reduces heart attack risk instead of increasing it?

If you're looking for a low-cost, effective prescription for health, look at your gardens, look at farmers' fields, look at the produce section of your grocery store. Plants are the best medicine you can find:

- Worried about obesity? Obesity and meat-eating are connected.[‡] Vegan diets help people lose weight.[§]
- Worried about diabetes? Vegetarians are less likely to have diabetes,[¶] and a plant-based diet can increase insulin sensitivity.[**]

[*]   Sinha R, Cross AJ, Graubard BI, Leitzmann MF, Schatzkin A. "Meat Intake and Mortality: A Prospective Study of over Half a Million People." Arch Intern Med. 2009 Mar 23;169(6): 562–71. DOI: http://dx.doi.org/10.1001/archinternmed.2009.6. [PMC free article] [PubMed]

[†]   "Report of the Dietary Guidelines Advisory Committee on the Dietary Guidelines for Americans, 2010: To the Secretary of Agriculture and the Secretary of Health and Human Services." Washington, DC: Agriculture Research Service, US Department of Agriculture, US Department of Health and Human Services, May 2010.

[‡]   Wang Y, Beydoun MA. "Meat Consumption Is Associated with Obesity and Central Obesity Among US Adults." Int J Obes (Lond) 2009 Jun;33(6): 621–8. DOI: http://dx.doi.org/10.1038/ijo.2009.45. [PMC free article] [PubMed]

[§]   Berkow SE, Barnard N. "Vegetarian Diets and Weight Status." Nutr Rev. 2006 Apr; 64(4): 175–88. DOI: http://dx.doi.org/10.1111/j.1753-4887.2006.tb00200.x. [PubMed]

[¶]   Vang A, Singh PN, Lee JW, Haddad EH, Brinegar CH. "Meats, Processed Meats, Obesity, Weight Gain and Occurrence of Diabetes Among Adults: Findings from Adventist Health Studies." Ann Nutr Metab. 2008; 52(2): 96–104. DOI: http://dx.doi.org/10.1159/000121365. [PubMed]

[**]   Barnard ND, Cohen J, Jenkins DJ, et al. "A Low-fat Vegan Diet Improves Glycemic Control and Cardiovascular Risk Factors in a Randomized Clinical Trial in Individuals with Type 2 Diabetes." Diabetes Care. August 2006; 29(8): 1777–83. DOI: http://dx.doi.org/10.2337/dc06-0606. [PubMed]

- Worried about your heart? Cardiovascular disease and atherosclerosis have both shown improvement in patients who have adopted plant-based diets.[*]

Now, are you ready to stop worrying? Want to prevent diabetes—or reverse the symptoms? Want to protect your heart? Want to burn more calories in less time?

You can. With plants. Compared to meat, plants . . .

- Are lower in calories
- Have more fiber
- Have fewer unhealthy fats

We all want to be healthier, and a plant-based diet is how to get there and stay there. Studies have shown that vegetarians eat *more* magnesium, potassium, iron, thiamin, riboflavin, folate, and vitamins and *less* total fat than nonvegetarians do.

Because of the health benefits of plant-based eating, the results of a plant-based diet are very different from those of a diet based on processed foods. Instead of sluggishness, an upset stomach, and a predisposition to obesity and diabetes, you'll have . . .

- heaps of energy
- a happy belly
- less heartburn
- balanced blood sugar levels
- a healthy weight
- a sense of contentment before, during, and after meals
- an improved mood

There is so much research that shows how good plants are for you and your family. Vegetarians live longer. They get cancer less frequently. They have fewer strokes. They don't suffer from heart disease as much. Vegans are also thinner! The benefits of a plant-based diet are numerous. Lower blood pressure, less diabetes, less asthma, and healthier cholesterol levels.

And if you love to eat—and you want a diet plan that lets you eat plenty without

---

[*]   Ornish D, Brown SE, Scherwitz LW, et al. "Can Lifestyle Changes Reverse Coronary Heart Disease? The Lifestyle Heart Trial." Lancet. 1990 Jul 21; 336(8708): 129–33. DOI: http://dx.doi.org/10.1016/0140-6736(90)91656-U. [PubMed]

feeling deprived—plants are the way to go. If you've ever had a look at the calorie count in fast-food meals, you know that they can have more than a thousand calories per entrée. That's a lot of calories with very little nutrition. Compare that to the plant-based meal you could have instead—five jumbo-size bowls of salad, a few bowls of fruit, and six avocados? Too much food to consume in one sitting!

Plants just give you more.

SKIP THE FRANKENFOODS. CHOOSE THE REAL FOODS

If you've done 22 Days before, you may have already read about "frankenfoods." What are frankenfoods? Like the original monster from books and movies, frankenfoods are created by scientists in a lab. Breakfast cereals coated in sugar; bright pink "meat" slices; sixteen-ounce or twenty-four-ounce beverages that are full of sugar and additives—all of these products that you think you are desiring, that you feel like you are craving, that you think will make you feel good, but will really make you feel terrible.

Too many people have become addicted to that crunch and to those false flavors, and the result? Huge profits for some companies, while their customers walk around sleepy, feeling sick, feeling bloated, feeling listless. Day by day, overprocessed foods, made in plants, are hurting us. They hurt our palates. They hurt our bodies. Short term, you feel nauseous or tired. Long term, illness creeps in. And if you don't exorcise the demons—with exercise and by changing your habits—those illnesses can move in for good and become chronic issues that threaten your long-term health and your life.

So what's next?

What's next is swapping the fake for the real, the imaginary for the ideal. With 22 Days, while you follow your menus of choice, while you learn to prep your kitchen so you can prep your meals efficiently as well as deliciously, you'll be reminding yourself what real food tastes like. If you've been eating too many processed foods, your taste buds have become accustomed to flat tastes, metallic tastes, and hyper-salty and sugary tastes. Your taste buds have become overwhelmed! Coax them back to life by giving yourself natural crunches, the delicate and spicy tastes of fresh herbs, the savory flavors of vegetables that have been simmering or roasting with plenty of garlic and onion. . . .

When you banish the frankenfoods, in a few days, you will see the change. That metallic taste is gone. That up-and-down spike and fall that come from added sugar are gone. Instead, you'll enjoy real foods, with the true sweetness of nature, the true rainbow of colors, the natural taste of foods that give you true health, that give you true energy, so you will look and feel your very best.

22 Days is about real, not fake. Grown, not made. Plants, not made in plants. Forget artificial flavors and colors and embrace REAL flavors and colors. 22 Days is a real-time solution, for real people, that you can really do—and really stick with.

There is nothing artificial about 22 Days. The results are very real.

FINDING TRUE COMFORT IN REAL FOOD

We want comfort foods to make us feel good. So we're offering you some new comfort foods here: foods that actually make you feel good, that make you feel truly satisfied.

We all want to eat well. We all want food that is delicious and satisfying. And we all get used to our comforts. Those cookies . . . those fast-food hamburgers . . . and that mile-high deli sandwich don't really offer comfort over the long term.

On the checklist of human wants and needs, we will all choose health over illness, energy over exhaustion, healthy weight loss over unhealthy weight gain, steady and sustainable weight instead of a lifetime on that seesaw of lose and gain, lose and gain, lose and gain.

Doesn't that sound like a kind of heaven? Where your stomach doesn't hurt after a feast. Where you don't experience regret after a meal. Where you don't wish hours later that you hadn't eaten so much or make empty promises to yourself never to do that again. But isn't that what our "comfort" foods give us? We've all had the experience of indulging in our favorite deep-fried, double-stuffed, triple-towered items—and the last thing they are is comfortable.

Really, those foods are discomfort foods.

If you eat processed foods regularly, if you rely on breads and grains that have been stripped of their nutrition, if you eat meat raised on hormones, meat in a can, or deli meat pumped up with extra sodium and flavor fillers—you are putting your health at risk. You're giving your energy levels a dip instead of a boost. You're eating too much salt. You're not getting enough nutrition. You are missing out on all of the benefits of a plant-based lifestyle. Including comfort!

As you begin your journey with 22 Days, you will try new foods and experience new flavors and some boosts for familiar favorites. Over time, you will find yourself craving different foods and different flavors from the ones you do now . . . perhaps the creamy Tahini Dressing, or the crispness of Cheezy Kale Chips or the spicy warmth of our Chana Masala Chickpeas. New comforts, real comforts, true comforts.

The crazy thing is that it's so simple! It's so easy! I'm not asking you to give up your happiness. I'm asking you to embrace happiness. I'm not asking you to stop enjoying yourself. I'm showing you how you can truly enjoy yourself, on every level, because when you eat plant-based foods, when you have that energy, when you stop wasting your thoughts on feeling BAD about your choices and experience that glow that comes from knowing you can feel GOOD about choosing meals that are GOOD for you—then you see how life can really be. Then you stop worrying about the rest of your life and start living the best of your life.

Because health is the most comfortable feeling there is.

FINDING THAT FEELING OF FULLNESS

Eating plants makes you more comfortable over the long run, and it also makes you feel better every single day, with every single meal. That's because so many people eat until they are too full. Eating too much at a meal leads to stomachaches, indigestion, exhaustion. Eating too much at every meal leads to weight gain and all of the issues that come along with extra pounds.

Getting back to that feeling of "I've had enough" is getting back to your most basic and natural self, before the world imposed all its ideas about food and eating on you. Think about it. If you've raised a child, you know that infants and young babies don't overeat. They don't stuff themselves silly and then get stomachaches. They don't eat when they are bored or when they are sad or angry. They eat when they are hungry. And when they are hungry, they will not hesitate to let you know! But no matter how hungry they were when they began their meal, as soon as they are full, they will cease eating. Even if it is delicious. Even if there is another course.

Babies naturally stop wanting food when their bodies have had enough. But somehow, as we get older, this all changes. Suddenly kids meet sugary foods, and then you see that light in their eyes as they want more, more, more. Suddenly they aren't thinking about how their bodies feel, because that sugar has overridden their natural instincts. Then they get a little older and they learn from adults that food is a reward, a destination, something we can turn to whenever we feel sad, feel scared. Hunger gets shoved to the corner; that natural association that having enough means stopping until later is broken. Instead, the new association changes, and it's no longer eat until you aren't hungry; it's just eat, as much as you want whenever you want.

And then we get a little older, and those habits start to catch up with us. Suddenly all those extra calories, that extra sugar, those missing nutrients start to have an effect, and if we don't go back to our natural healthful habits (stopping when you are full), our new habits (unbuckling your belt and mindless eating) lead to obesity. Lead to diabetes. Lead to chronic illnesses that could have been avoided if we could just reintroduce ourselves to our natural way of eating.

If you have been overeating, 22 Days can reintroduce you to the joys of restraint.

If you've been using food to cover up your feelings, 22 Days can help you remember what it feels like to feel GREAT.

If you've been stuck on the up-and-down roller coaster of sugar abuse, 22 Days can remind you how delicious and invigorating sweet fruits, juices, and smoothies can be and how eating plants can stabilize your blood sugar and your moods.

You will find success if you invest the time to buy fresh produce. If you invest the energy to prepare loving and healthful meals for you and your family. And become very, very skilled at stopping when you are full.

WHY I INCLUDE CALORIE COUNTS

If you're a *22-Day Revolution* regular, you'll notice that this volume has something added: calorie counts. Usually, I don't include calorie counts because I want people to know what full feels like instead of relying on mathematics. In this case, I'm asking you to use the math as a tool to help you maximize your grasp on what satisfaction feels like.

Too many people connect the idea of "fullness" with the feeling of "bursting." The sensation that you might explode is NOT what fullness feels like! Full is a quiet satisfaction when your body has been given the right amount of energy for the moment. My hope is that by seeing the calorie count, eating an appropriate amount of energy, and then experiencing what that amount of energy feels like in your body, you will begin to understand what full *really* feels like.

At the beginning, if you are used to overstuffing your system, full might feel like you still want more. Like you are still hungry. So give it a moment. Give it time. It's going to take more than one meal to reset your physical sensors. Have you ever had a car light go on when you know there is enough gas in the car or when you know you have just had your tires inflated? Sometimes the light means there is an issue with your car's light sensors, not with the gas tank or the tires.

What I'm suggesting here is that sometimes when you want to keep eating after you've had your portion, there is nothing wrong with your gas tank. It is your sensor—the way you experience that feeling—that needs resetting. Once you have become accustomed to eating smaller portions, with the right amount of calories for your body, your sensors will reset. You will feel what full really feels like—and the truth is that full feels like nothing much at all. Full is a quiet feeling, and the calorie counts can help you get just the right amount of food.

You can use this enhanced awareness at every point in your journey. Whether you are just beginning or resetting your system, whether you are here to lose forty pounds or twenty pounds or two pounds, keeping your attention on how you truly feel will be a useful guide to you. If you can't feel it yet, don't worry—you can do the math! You can use the numbers to make sure you are working toward your goals.

The calories are provided as a guide to help you gauge how much food your body actually needs for you to feel energized. Along with the adjustable menus, understanding calories will help you grasp how simple it is to calibrate your daily intake, just by having less at night if you have more in the morning, just by adding a snack if you need more energy, or by not having dessert if you've had a snack.

And as time goes on, you will find that if you overeat at any meal, you will notice the too full feeling, even without having a calorie count nearby. Even without seeing the calories, you will know you've overdone it. That is a success in and of itself.

WHEN EATING IS IN BALANCE, WEIGHT COMES INTO BALANCE

A balanced diet is one in which the three macronutrients—carbohydrates, proteins, and fats—are all present and accounted for in the proper amounts. Skimping on one or the other doesn't help you; having too much of them doesn't help you; the best way to help yourself achieve your best is by balancing carbs, proteins, and fats. And that balance has a ratio of 80-10-10. This means that MOST of your nutrition and energy will come from carbohydrates, SOME will come from protein, and SOME will come from fat: 80-10-10. (This may vary slightly from person to person.)

80% carbohydrates
10% proteins
10% fat

CARBOHYDRATES

High in fiber, with the power to fuel your whole body, including (and especially) your brain, carbs will make up 80 percent of your daily food intake. When complex carbs are broken down, you get glucose, which your whole body uses as an energy source.

You'll be eating carbohydrates in the form of fruits, vegetables, grains, and legumes (and avoiding their simpler, not-as-great-for-you cousins, like pizza and cake and anything made of white flour).

PROTEIN

Plants can give you all the protein you need, even if you're an athlete. Protein builds your muscles and helps with tissue repair. All of your cells rely on the protein you eat for amino acids, the building blocks of protein. Your body can make some amino acids but not others; you can get the ones you need, called "essential amino acids," from plant sources like quinoa, nuts, seeds, and combinations of grains and legumes. Rice and beans, corn and beans, rice and lentils—all of these deliver the protein you need to live and thrive.

FATS

Fats come in different types, and some of them are exactly what your body needs for health. When you think about fats, think unsaturated: monounsaturated, polyunsaturated, and omega-3s. Those are the fats that will be in the 22-Day recipes. What we're skipping are saturated fats and trans fats and the health dangers that accompany them.

Remember: Foods with trans fats (like margarine and processed snacks) are to be avoided. Foods with saturated fats (like meats, lard, and butter) are to be avoided or limited in the case of saturated fats found in some plants.

With *The 22-Day Revolution*, we craft balanced menus, and you buy your produce and prepare your meals. While you're eating, you can relax and know that you are eating a balanced and healthy ratio of nutrients, with the right amount of fats, carbohydrates, and proteins, plus all the vitamins, minerals, and phytonutrients your body needs.

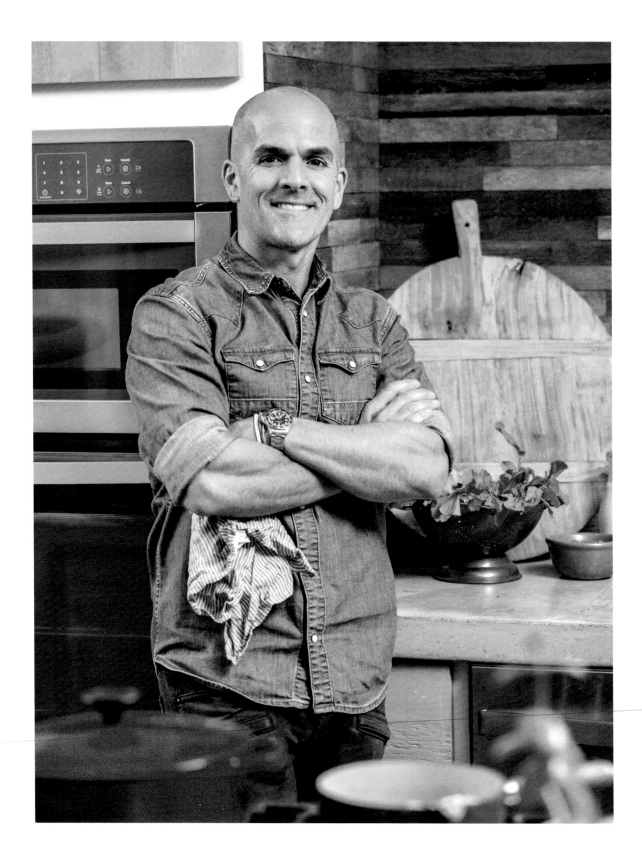

BUILD YOUR OWN 22-DAY PROGRAM

WHICH 22-DAY PROGRAM IS RIGHT FOR YOU?

There are four new, customizable programs included in the *22-Day Revolution Cookbook*: two for losing weight and two for maintaining or building muscle. All of our plans have flexible menus based on your eating style and a balance of 80 percent carbs, 10 percent protein, and 10 percent fat.

These programs are adaptable to you. We don't live in a one-size-fits-all world. We all have our own busy schedules and our own ways of doing things. My-way-or-the-highway programs don't work for long. Programs that don't take YOU into account can't work for long, because you are what makes a program work. You are the energy behind the machine. You are the power that lights the way of your transformation.

Of course, we all need guidance to succeed, and what ensures our success is guidance that works with our needs.

I see it all the time. I have heard countless stories from people who have tried and failed at one, two, three, a hundred programs before they found their way to 22 Days. They start a program because they get a glimpse of something better, of something powerful, and they want a part of it. And then all of those beautiful feelings, hopes and efforts are dashed when the programs are too hard, or they don't work in the real world or with real lives.

That's the beauty of 22 Days. With 22 Days, you're in charge.

With every program, as you accustom yourself to the portions and the plant-based meals, as your body gets used to how it feels to be truly full and not overstuffed and uncomfortable, you will find a sense of peace and balance.

Finding the right program helps short-term changes become lifelong habits.

OUR FOUR FLEXIBLE PROGRAMS

Where you begin depends on where you're at right now. You'll start with FAST TRACK if you have a lot of weight to lose. LIGHT AND BRIGHT is for weight loss, for those last stubborn pounds or a quick reset. NIRVANA is for maintenance and daily healthy living. ATHLETE'S ADVANTAGE is a short-term training menu.

FAST TRACK ▶ If you want to lose twenty, thirty, forty pounds or more, begin with FAST TRACK. FAST TRACK is your fast weight-loss plan and hard-core reset. FAST TRACK will help you use the benefits of plants to care for and nourish your body as you shed fat and build muscle by working out.

- If you have ten to fifty pounds to lose
- If you are tired of trying diets that don't work for the long term
- If you have big goals and are ready to achieve them
- If you have a wedding, a graduation, a black-tie event, or a red-carpet event to attend

FAST TRACK will help you shed weight quickly. Once you've reached your FAST TRACK goals, you're ready for LIGHT AND BRIGHT.

LIGHT AND BRIGHT ▶ If you want to lose up to ten pounds, try LIGHT AND BRIGHT, which helps you lose the weight while you rev up your energy and your vitality. LIGHT AND BRIGHT is your weight-loss and reset plan. If you're ready for LIGHT AND BRIGHT, you:

- Are just beginning 22 Days, and you only have ten pounds to go
- Have already lost weight with 22 Days and you're ready for more
- Are a graduate of the FAST TRACK program
- Are ready for a reset

LIGHT AND BRIGHT will help you get rid of those last stubborn pounds. Once you've reached your LIGHT AND BRIGHT goals, you're ready for NIRVANA.

NIRVANA ▶ You're living the best time of your life! Now that you're (pretty) happy with your weight, you want to stay there. Once we reach NIRVANA, why go back? NIRVANA is your maintenance plan, so you can keep on feeling great by continuing to do what got you here: eating plants. If you're ready for NIRVANA, you:

- Have already done your 22 Days and lost your desired weight
- Are looking to maintain your current weight and get all the benefits of plants
- Are looking to transition to a plant-based menu
- Don't need to lose weight but want to increase your consciousness and awareness

The NIRVANA plan is your maintenance and well-being plan, designed for sustainability. If you've reached your goals and you want to stay there, the NIRVANA program will help you keep eating plants, so you can eat well, live well, and be well. If you're at your fittest, or close to it, and you're about to test your fitness with an endurance event, use the ATHLETE'S ADVANTAGE menu while you train.

ATHLETE'S ADVANTAGE ▶ You're nearing your goals and you want to take on the challenge of a 10K run or a triathlon. Or you're an athlete who's heard about the edge that eating plants can give you while you're climbing, biking, running, or competing. Our training menu provides extra energy for those times when you're heading for the peak, the ribbon, the edge of the horizon. ATHLETE'S ADVANTAGE is for those who are participating in high-intensity or long-duration athletics and need extra carbs for energy and extra protein for muscle repair. If you're ready for ATHLETE'S ADVANTAGE, you:

- Are at your goal weight or close, and you are in training for an event
- Are an athlete curious about the advantage that plant-based meals can give you
- Already run fast and want to run faster

The ATHLETE'S ADVANTAGE plan is a short-term menu for athletes only. Only use the ATHLETE'S ADVANTAGE menu if your goal is ENDURANCE, not WEIGHT LOSS. After your event, return to the NIRVANA program.

RESETS

I'm a big fan of resets. Of course, in an ideal world, we'd all be eating well every single day. But that's not how the real world works. So if you've fallen off the track—use a reset to get back on. No matter how good our intentions are, sometimes we fall off the wagon, lose the path, miss a beat. A reset gives you a chance to examine your habits and the way your body feels after meals, and to consider the foods you've been giving yourself. With a reset, you can get conscious, get aware, and get back on track.

HOW TO USE THE PROGRAMS

With every program, you'll be eating three meals a day and, in some, either a snack or dessert. Using the guidelines for each program, you choose your meals from two categories—LIGHT or INDULGENT, mixing and matching the recipes so you can always have the food you're in the mood for when you're in the mood for it. Light breakfast, meals, snacks, and desserts contain fewer calories to fuel your weight-loss goals, while the indulgent options are heartier and nutrient dense. The following shows the amount of calories that you will find for each category level:

LIGHT

- Breakfast: < 400 calories
- Meals (Lunch and Dinner): < 300 calories
- Snacks: < 150 calories
- Desserts: ≤150 calories

INDULGENT

- Breakfast: > 400 calories
- Meals (Lunch and Dinner): ≥ 300 calories
- Snacks: ≥ 150 calories
- Desserts: > 150 calories

For each week of your 22-Day program, eat according to the plans below, choosing meals from the light or indulgent categories. It is up to you on how the days are ordered throughout the week. These programs are designed to fit your particular goals and can be followed exactly. Or if you choose, you can follow any combination that best suits your lifestyle.

Within the four programs—FAST TRACK, LIGHT AND BRIGHT, NIRVANA, and ATHLETE'S ADVANTAGE—there are a combination of suggested light and indulgent meals for a particular amount of days of the week. All recipes are organized within each meal category—breakfast, lunch and dinner, snacks, and desserts—and are color-coded: green for light and orange for indulgent. Use the colors as a guide when selecting a combination of light and indulgent meals within each category to meet the goals for each program. This system is meant to be flexible, save time, and help you stay focused and be consistent and successful.

FAST TRACK ▶

You've used the 22-Day program and you want more so you can lose more weight. Or you're new to the program and you want to get started here and now. Great. The fast-track program is designed so you can get the most out of your meals and still lose weight as fast as you want to. Plant-based foods are so powerful, so full of nutrients, so beneficial for your body, your organs, your muscles, your skin—by eating plant-based for twenty-two days, you will revolutionize the way you look and feel and completely change your relationship with food and your body.

For each week of your 22-Day program, eat according to the plan below, choosing meals from the Level 1 Light or Level 2 Indulgent categories.

- On 3 days, choose Level 1 meals for breakfast, lunch, and dinner. No snack.
- On 2 days, choose Level 1 meals for breakfast and dinner, and choose a heartier Level 2 option for lunch. No snack.
- On 2 days, choose Level 2 meals for breakfast and lunch, and choose Level 1 options for dinner and snack or dessert.

DAYS	BREAKFAST LEVEL	LUNCH LEVEL	DINNER LEVEL	SNACK/DESSERT LEVEL
3	LIGHT	LIGHT	LIGHT	X
2	LIGHT	INDULGENT	LIGHT	X
2	INDULGENT	INDULGENT	LIGHT	LIGHT

LIGHT AND BRIGHT ▶

You may be new to the program and just need to shed a few pounds . . . or you've been using the 22-Day program and you're ready for some new flavors. Light and bright is for people who want full-on nutrition, satisfaction, and the best-tasting meals and snacks while they get all the health benefits of eating plant-based foods, from weight loss to maximum energy to improving heart health and lowering risks for diabetes and other illnesses.

For each week of your 22-Day program, eat according to the plan below, choosing meals from the Level 1 Light or Level 2 Indulgent categories.

- On 3 days, choose Level 1 meals for breakfast and dinner, and choose a heartier Level 2 option for lunch. No snack.
- On 2 days, choose Level 2 meals for breakfast and lunch, and choose a lighter Level 1 option for dinner and for a snack or dessert.
- On 2 days, choose Level 2 meals for breakfast, lunch and dinner, and choose a Level 2 snack or dessert.

DAYS	BREAKFAST LEVEL	LUNCH LEVEL	DINNER LEVEL	SNACK/DESSERT LEVEL
3	LIGHT	INDULGENT	LIGHT	X
2	INDULGENT	INDULGENT	LIGHT	LIGHT
2	INDULGENT	INDULGENT	INDULGENT	INDULGENT

NIRVANA ▶

Stay strong and focused by tuning up your body with a great workout, and tuning up your nutrition with plant-based meals. This maintenance program is about sustaining health, keeping your food and your body in balance, and continuing to enjoy your mealtime, your healthy body, and your life, day by day.

For each week of your 22-Day program, eat according to the plan below, choosing meals from the Level 1 Light or Level 2 Indulgent categories.

- On 5 days, choose Level 2 meals for breakfast and lunch, and choose a lighter Level 1 option for dinner and for a snack or dessert.
- On 2 days, choose a Level 1 meal for breakfast and Level 2 options for lunch and dinner. Enjoy a Level 2 snack or dessert.

DAYS	BREAKFAST LEVEL	LUNCH LEVEL	DINNER LEVEL	SNACK/DESSERT LEVEL
5	INDULGENT	INDULGENT	LIGHT	LIGHT
2	LIGHT	INDULGENT	INDULGENT	INDULGENT

ATHLETE'S ADVANTAGE ▶

Yes, athletes can thrive on a plant-based diet. I eat a plant-based diet, and I am always pushing myself to achieve new goals and training my clients. Muscles are made of protein, and energy comes from carbohydrates and fat, and a plant-based diet delivers ample amounts of the things your body needs. Training for a 10K, a marathon, or a triple threat? We got you. Carb-loading before a big race? No problem. The training menu offers ample energy when you've got a trail to conquer, a bike to own, an ocean to swim, or a road to burn, no matter how many miles you have to go.

For each week of your 22-Day program, eat according to the plan below, choosing meals from the Level 1 Light or Level 2 Indulgent categories.

- On 5 days, choose Level 2 meals for breakfast, lunch and dinner. Enjoy a Level 2 snack or dessert.
- On 2 days, choose a Level 2 meal for breakfast and lunch, and a Level 1 option for dinner. Select a Level 1 snack or dessert.

DAYS	BREAKFAST LEVEL	LUNCH LEVEL	DINNER LEVEL	SNACK/DESSERT LEVEL
5	INDULGENT	INDULGENT	INDULGENT	INDULGENT
2	INDULGENT	INDULGENT	LIGHT	LIGHT

PLAN FOR SUCCESS

Stock Your Pantry, Write Your Shopping List, Prepare Your Kitchen

FARM TO PANTRY

Farm to table is a big deal these days; you can't read a food magazine or make a restaurant reservation without hearing those words. Eating farm to table at home—or garden to table, or farmers' market to table—begins before you ever get to the table. It begins in your kitchen and your pantry.

Getting your space ready to support you as you make small changes that will transform you in a big way is the first step in making a healthier life a possibility and a reality. So let's clean up your kitchen. And I don't mean washing the floors (but please do, if they need it). I mean shedding the unhealthy foods so you can shed those pounds. The sooner it's out of the house, the sooner you can stop being tempted. The sooner your shelves are full of healthy choices, the sooner you can easily make healthier choices.

RESET

Throw out all of the processed foods. Get rid of the sugary foods. You know what I'm talking about. You know what I mean. Just do it. The cookie dough in the fridge, the cookies on the counter, that old bologna—get rid of it.

If it has ADDED SUGAR, CORN SYRUP, ARTIFICIAL SWEETENERS, WHITE FLOUR, DAIRY, EGGS, or MEAT, get it out of your kitchen.

RESTOCK

Once your kitchen is clean, go shopping for the kinds of food you really want to be craving.

You'll want to shop for organic produce: fresh fruits and fresh vegetables.

You'll want to purchase healthy pantry items like organic grains and cereals, like nuts and seeds. Replace that sugary peanut butter with fresh almond butter. Get tomato sauce without sugar. The same goes for salad dressing.

We've included a pantry list to help you, and you'll want to be shopping weekly to make sure you have the freshest produce for your menus. Remember not to shop hungry—eat a snack first! Hungry eyes are big eyes. And be generous with yourself. If there's a fruit you want to try, try it. If there's a new kind of vegetable, buy it and then figure out how to cook it later. Try new things. Try it all! There are new favorites hiding behind every corner of the produce section. . . .

WHY I EAT ORGANIC

I eat organic produce because I know that traditional farming uses more than four hundred different kinds of pesticides. And pesticides do damage! How crazy is it that some of us are eating fruits and vegetables because we want to be healthier, and the way they are grown is actually putting us at risk for diseases. If you avoid foods that are high in pesticides, you may be able to reduce the risk of some diseases, which include Alzheimer's and Parkinson's, both very serious illnesses in this country today. When I go food shopping, I look for organic, GMO-free produce so I am sure that my family is getting the best available.

According to legal definitions, organic foods are grown without artificial pesticides and herbicides, growth hormones, genetically modified organisms (GMOs), or synthetic fertilizers. That way I'm getting more of what I want—nutrition—and less of what I don't—poisons.

POWERFUL PANTRY STAPLES

Having staples in your pantry makes it so much easier when trying to prepare meals, especially with a limited amount of time.

- **LEGUMES:** Studies have shown that adding a minimum of a half cup of cooked legumes six days a week may reduce the risk of type 2 diabetes, many types of cardiovascular disease, and several types of cancer.

  When time permits, cooking beans from scratch is a great idea, but when you are pressed for time, it's nice to have cooked boxed or BPA-free cans on hand. Having both, dried and canned, makes it easier when preparing meals.

  Legumes are superior sources of protein.
    - adzuki (1 cup cooked equals 17 grams protein)
    - black beans (1 cup cooked equals 15.2 grams protein)
    - garbanzo beans (1 cup equals 14.5 grams protein)
    - great northern beans (navy beans) (1 cup cooked equals 14.7 grams protein)
    - white kidney beans (cannellini) (1 cup cooked equals 17.4 grams protein)
    - split peas (contain 16.4 grams protein)
    - lentils (1 cup lentils contain 17.9 grams protein)

- **NUTS:** almonds, cashews, peanuts, pecans, pine nuts, pistachios, walnuts

- **GRAINS:** brown rice, millet, oats

- **SEEDS** *(used frequently in this book)*: quinoa, chia (including milled chia), flax (including flax meal), hemp, pumpkin, and sesame

- **NUT BUTTERS:** almond, cashew, pecan, pine nut, pistachio, walnut

- **FROZEN FRUITS:** bananas, blackberries, blueberries, mangoes, pineapples, raspberries, strawberries (we like to buy them fresh and organic, and whatever we don't eat by the end of the week, we freeze)

- **DRIED FRUIT:** cranberries, dates, goji berries, raisins, golden berries

- **FROZEN FOOD:** veggies, fruit, shredded coconut

- **DRIED HERBS AND SPICES:** Stocking up on dried herbs and spices makes it easier when preparing recipes. Try having these on hand: basil, cayenne pepper, chili powder, cinnamon (ground), coriander (ground), cumin (ground), curry powder, dill weed, garlic powder, ginger (ground), nutmeg, onion powder, oregano leaves, paprika, parsley flakes, red pepper (crushed flakes), rosemary, smoked paprika, thyme, turmeric (ground).

- **SAUCES, SEASONINGS, AND CONDIMENTS:** The following is a list of some of our favorites that are used often in our recipes. Feel free to have on hand any of your favorites that you might want to include in your meal. Apple cider vinegar, balsamic vinegar, coconut vinegar, brown rice vinegar, barbecue sauce and ketchup (even though we have our own version for homemade), Dijon mustard, nutritional yeast, olives, sea salt, coconut aminos, tomato paste

- **SWEETENERS:** applesauce (unsweetened), coconut palm sugar, powdered natural sugar (made from unrefined sugar), pure maple syrup, coconut water

- **FLOURS FOR BAKING AND COOKING AND OTHER ESSENTIALS:** almond flour, millet flour, arrowroot flour, vegan chocolate chips, cocoa powder, oat flour, quinoa flour, brown rice flour, pure vanilla extract, tapioca flour, milled chia seeds, flax meal, dry active yeast, baking soda, baking powder

THE POWER OF PLANNING

Planning ahead reduces stress in the kitchen and is the most effective strategy for maintaining a healthy diet. Try planning your meals for the next few days or a week ahead, and consider preparing enough to have leftovers. This way you can plan how to use them, reducing the amount of food you waste. Did you know the average American tosses away about 25 percent of food and beverages purchased? Planning ahead can help reduce this drastically!

Some simple recipes to consider for the week are baked goods, muesli, granola, cashew cheese, salad dressings, walnut meat, quinoa, brown rice, and beans, which can save you a lot of time in the kitchen. For example, it's nice to have in the freezer nutritious baked goods, which can be reheated for a quick breakfast, or seeded whole-grain bread, which can be toasted and topped simply with cashew cheese or a nut butter. Or try keeping a batch of frozen veggie burgers to pop in the oven and enjoy with mixed greens or sliced avocado and tomato. Another important tip: Having pre-washed fruits and vegetables can be very helpful. Some fruits, such as berries, shouldn't be washed until you're ready to use them because they spoil easily, but for most fruits and vegetables, consider buying prewashed vegetables or washing your vegetables before storing them in the refrigerator.

Just remember to strategically plan in order to achieve your personal goals, and you'll be on your way to the best version of you!

THE 22-DAY REVOLUTION COOKBOOK

NO MATTER WHAT YOU THINK you love to eat, you can learn to love eating plants. As soon as you take those first steps, you'll see the enormous benefits right away. When you put good food into your body, you feel better about yourself. There's a certain kind of empowerment that comes from eating better, from feeling better, from looking better.

The effects of eating a plant-based diet are beneficial for health and wellness—and that includes every area of your life. When you feel great, and when your body is buzzing with the energy and nutrition from a plant-based diet, everything is easier.

Developing the habit of eating plants gives you the energy to deal with life—the energy to live your life in a positive, kind, and compassionate way and to make the right choices for yourself so you can be your healthiest, inside and out.

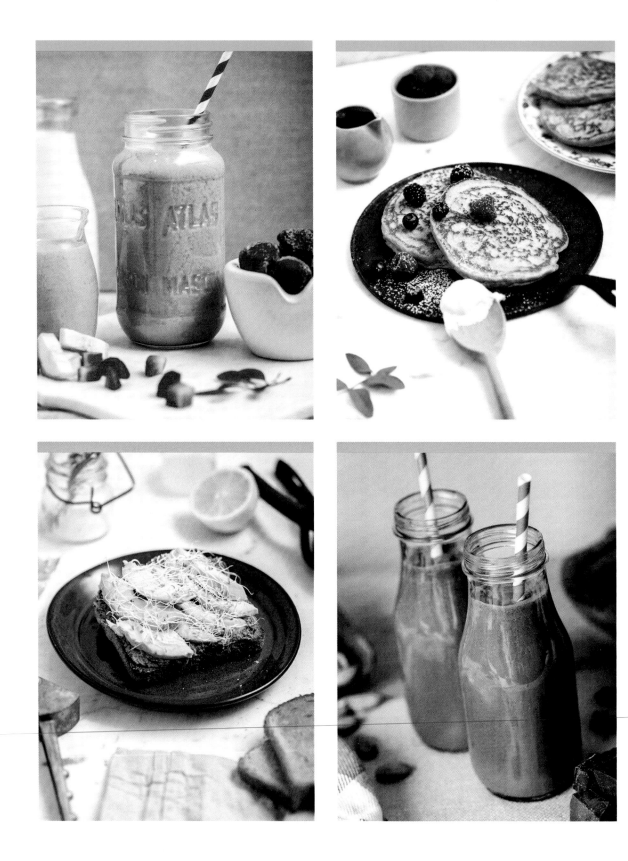

BREAKFAST

BREAKFAST ISN'T REALLY THE most important meal of the day. It's the FIRST important meal of the day. For me and my family, breakfast is the time when we celebrate a new day together.

My favorite breakfast recipes are Banana and Almond Butter Breakfast Quinoa and Avocado Tomato Bruschetta because it gives me the energy I need to start my day and sets the tone for lunch and dinner.

Smoothies and juices are great first meals, especially when you are rushing out the door. The main difference between a smoothie and a juice is the amount of fiber you're consuming. Smoothies retain the pulp from fruits and vegetables and provide a filling source of vitamins, which keeps you feeling full longer.

Juicing is a great way to heal, renew, and rebuild your immune system, while detoxifying and nurturing your body with antioxidants, enzymes, vitamins, and minerals. It's also an easy way to increase your daily servings of fruits and vegetables.

The vitamins and minerals from juicing are more easily absorbed on an empty stomach; therefore, starting your day with a freshly made juice is the best way to reap all the nutritional benefits.

Baked goods are also very filling and nutritious. For breads that are easy to handle and bursting with flavor, let them cool completely and store (overnight) untouched in an airtight container before slicing. Not only do the flavors of the sweet and savory breads intensify this way, but also the crust softens, making it easier to slice and preventing the bread from crumbling and falling apart.

For nut-free options, try substituting the almond flour with oat or brown rice flour. In most of the recipes that contain nuts, the nuts can be replaced by seeds or more flour. The taste and texture might change, but the overall flavor is still delicious.

We've included easy Light Level 1 options like super smoothies and juices for quick and delicious breakfasts when you're on the run, and heartier Indulgent Level 2 breakfasts you can use for delectable weekend brunches—and kids will love them too!

These recipes are quick to fix and make you and your family feel satisfied. Starting your morning with a healthy meal also gives you the energy you need for the rest of your busy and wonderful day.

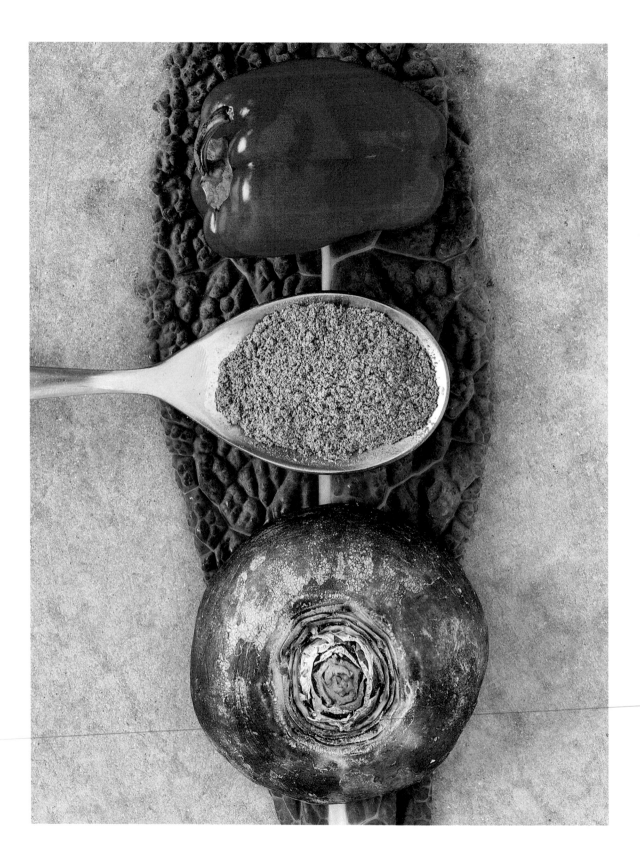

LEVEL 1

LIGHT BREAKFASTS

(UNDER 400 CALORIES)

There are so many light breakfast options that may surprise you—from sweet and satisfying Cinnamon Apple Bread and Lemon Chia Muffins to some of my favorite, filling smoothies like the Berry Mango Hemp Smoothie.

Smoothies and juices are a fun and easy way to add more greens and powerful antioxidants to your diet. Have fun trying different combinations and bring your kids into the mix by letting them experiment. Make smoothies and juices at home for a nutrient-dense option in the morning or at any time of the day. Whenever possible, avoid commercially bought bottled smoothies, which are often loaded with sugars and devoid of nutrients.

LIGHT

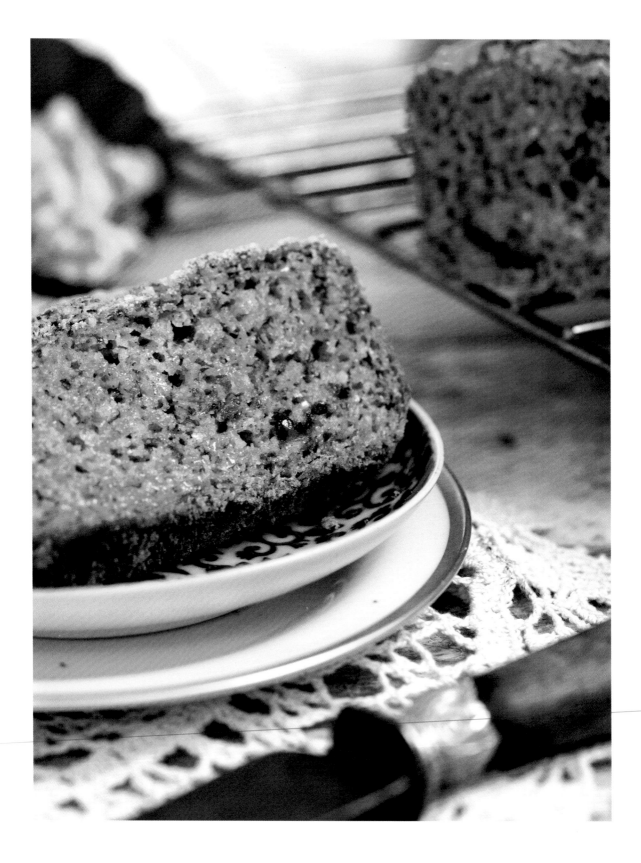

BANANA BREAD

▶ **NO OIL** ▶ **REFINED SUGAR-FREE**

PREP TIME: 10 min
COOK TIME: 50 min
TOTAL TIME: 60 min

MAKES ABOUT 12 SLICES

My mom always had a loaf of fresh Cuban bread in our home while we were growing up, so naturally I grew up eating lots of bread, but unfortunately not the good kind. I gave up most commercial breads years ago because of the terrible ingredients that go into them, but that doesn't mean I don't love or enjoy bread anymore. My wife, Marilyn, has created tons of amazing recipes, but this is one of my favorite. Banana bread that is both filling and delicious without weighing you down with unhealthy ingredients.

INGREDIENTS:

1 ripe banana, mashed

¾ cup sweetened vanilla almond milk

5 tablespoons maple syrup

2 tablespoons applesauce

1 teaspoon vanilla extract

½ teaspoon apple cider vinegar

½ cup brown rice flour

½ cup oat flour

½ cup tapioca and/or arrowroot flour

½ cup almond flour

1 tablespoon flax meal

1 tablespoon ground chia seeds

2 teaspoons baking powder

½ teaspoon baking soda

1 teaspoon ground cinnamon

¼ cup chopped walnuts

PREPARATION:

1. Preheat oven to 350F. Lightly grease a small (8" x 4") loaf pan or line it with parchment paper.

2. In a bowl, mix together the mashed banana and all other wet ingredients and set aside.

3. In another bowl, whisk together all dry ingredients except the walnuts.

4. Pour the wet ingredients over the dry and stir to combine well. Fold in the walnuts.

5. Pour the mixture into the loaf pan. Bake for about 50 minutes or until a toothpick inserted into the center of the loaf comes out clean. Remove the pan from the oven and let it cool before transferring the loaf from the pan to a wire rack. Cool completely, then slice, and serve!

Recipe continues

TIP: For muffins, simply pour the batter into a lightly greased or lined standard 12-cup muffin pan and bake for about 20 to 24 minutes at 350F. Leftovers can be stored at room temperature in an airtight container for up to a few days, in the refrigerator for up to a week, or in the freezer, in freezer bags layered with parchment paper, for up to a few months.

NOTE: Like most quick breads, make sure to cool completely to prevent crumbling. For best results, wrap the cooled bread in plastic wrap or store in an airtight container for several hours or overnight before slicing. Quick breads taste and slice best when enjoyed a day after baking.

PER SERVING: 135 calories, 2 grams protein, 23 grams carbohydrates, 5 grams total fat

CINNAMON APPLE BREAD LOAF

▶ **NO OIL**   ▶ **REFINED SUGAR-FREE**

PREP TIME: 10 min

COOK TIME: 50 min

TOTAL TIME: 60 min

MAKES ABOUT 12 SLICES

There's something about the aroma of a freshly baked loaf with cinnamon and apple that is so warm and comforting! This oil-free loaf is another guiltless sweet bread that's a favorite in our home. I find that because of the natural oils from the almond meal and walnuts, it's not necessary to add extra oil, but that's completely optional. Coconut oil is a great option, shown to have many health benefits. Adding coconut oil will give the loaf a subtle taste of coconut while adding extra moisture to the loaf. I've baked this bread both ways, and I love it either way!

INGREDIENTS:

1 cup unsweetened applesauce

½ cup sweetened vanilla almond milk or other nondairy milk

⅓ cup maple syrup—add 1 tablespoon, if you prefer a slightly sweeter loaf

1 teaspoon vanilla extract

½ teaspoon apple cider vinegar

½ cup brown rice flour

½ cup oat flour

½ cup tapioca and/or arrowroot flour

½ cup almond flour

1 tablespoon flax meal

1 tablespoon ground chia seeds

2 teaspoons baking powder

½ teaspoon baking soda

1 teaspoon ground cinnamon

1 small Fuji apple, peeled, cored, and chopped

¼ cup chopped walnuts

PREPARATION:

1. Preheat oven to 350F and lightly grease a small (8" x 4") loaf pan or line it with parchment paper.

2. In a bowl, mix together the wet ingredients.

3. In another bowl, whisk together the dry ingredients, except for the apple and walnuts.

4. Pour the wet ingredients over the dry and stir. Fold in the apples and walnuts.

5. Pour into the loaf pan and bake for 50 minutes or until a toothpick inserted into the center of the loaf comes out clean. Remove the pan from the oven and let it cool before transferring the loaf from the pan to a wire rack. Cool completely (at least 1 hour), then slice, and serve!

Recipe continues

TIP: Leftovers can be stored at room temperature in an airtight container for up to a few days, in the refrigerator for up to a week, or in the freezer, in freezer bags layered with parchment paper, for up to a few months.

NOTE: Like most quick breads, make sure to cool completely to prevent crumbling. For best results, wrap the cooled bread in plastic wrap or store in an airtight container for several hours or overnight before slicing. Quick breads taste and slice best when enjoyed a day after baking.

PER SERVING: 150 calories, 3 grams protein, 26 grams carbohydrates, 5 grams total fat

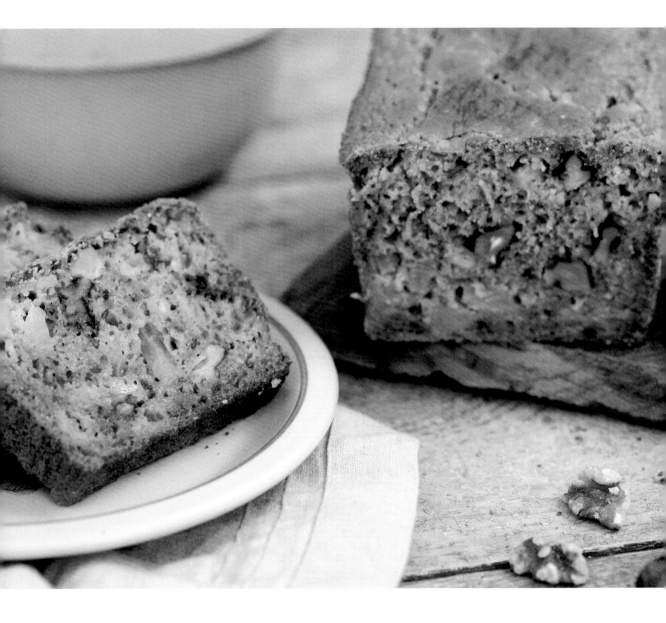

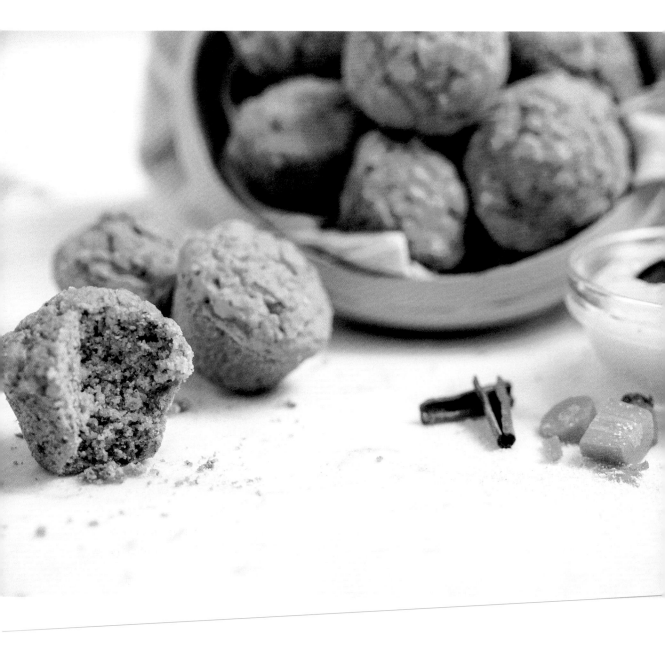

CARROT WALNUT MINI MUFFINS

▶ **NO OIL** ▶ **REFINED SUGAR-FREE**

PREP TIME: 10 min

COOK TIME: 22 min

TOTAL TIME: 32 min

MAKES 24 MUFFINS

We love making muffins, and these might just be our boys' favorite. Light and fluffy with carrots and walnuts, which are loaded with vitamins, minerals, and phytonutrients, these muffins are great for breakfast or as a snack any time of day.

INGREDIENTS:

¾ cup sweetened vanilla almond milk

½ cup maple syrup

2 tablespoons applesauce

½ teaspoon vanilla extract

½ teaspoon apple cider vinegar

¾ cup brown rice flour

¾ cup oat flour

½ cup almond flour

1 tablespoon flax meal

1 tablespoon ground chia seeds

1½ teaspoons baking powder

½ teaspoon baking soda

½ teaspoon ground cinnamon

1 cup finely grated carrots, not packed

¼ cup chopped walnuts

PREPARATION:

1. Preheat oven to 350F and lightly grease a 24-cup mini muffin pan or line it with paper liners.

2. In a bowl, mix together all liquid ingredients and set aside.

3. In another bowl, whisk together all dry ingredients except for the carrots and walnuts.

4. Pour the liquid ingredients over the dry and stir to combine. Fold in the carrots and walnuts.

5. Evenly pour the mixture into muffin cups and bake for 18 to 22 minutes or until a toothpick inserted into the center of a cupcake comes out clean.

6. Remove the pan from the oven and let it cool before transferring muffins to a wire rack.

TIP: You can also use a standard 12-cup muffin pan and bake at 350F for 20 to 24 minutes. Leftovers can be stored at room temperature in an airtight container for a few days, in the refrigerator for up to a week, or in the freezer, in freezer bags layered with parchment paper, for up to a few months.

PER SERVING: 70 calories, 2 grams protein, 12 grams carbohydrates, 2 grams total fat

ZUCCHINI BREAD LOAF

▶ **NO OIL** ▶ **REFINED SUGAR-FREE**

PREP TIME: 10 min

COOK TIME: 50 min

TOTAL TIME: 60 min

MAKES ABOUT 12 SLICES

This zucchini bread is a fun variation of our sweet bread with some veggies to kick up the nutrient density.

INGREDIENTS:

½ cup sweetened vanilla almond milk

½ cup plus 1 tablespoon maple syrup

2 tablespoons applesauce

1 teaspoon vanilla extract

½ teaspoon apple cider vinegar

½ cup brown rice flour

½ cup oat flour

½ cup tapioca and/or arrowroot flour

½ cup almond flour

2 tablespoons ground chia seeds or flax meal

2 teaspoons baking powder

½ teaspoon baking soda

1 teaspoon ground cinnamon

1 cup finely grated zucchini, loosely packed

PREPARATION:

1. Preheat oven to 350F and lightly grease a small (8" x 4") loaf pan or line it with parchment paper.

2. In a bowl, mix together the wet ingredients and set aside.

3. In another bowl, whisk together the dry ingredients, except for the grated zucchini.

4. Pour the wet ingredients over the dry and stir. Fold in the zucchini.

5. Pour the mixture into the loaf pan and bake for 50 minutes or until a toothpick inserted into the center of the loaf comes out clean. Remove the pan from the oven and let it cool before transferring the loaf from the pan to a wire rack. Cool completely (at least 1 or 2 hours), then slice, and serve!

TIP: Leftovers can be stored in an airtight container at room temperature for up to a few days, in the refrigerator for up to a week, or in the freezer, layered with parchment paper in freezer bags, for up to a few months.

NOTE: Like most quick breads, make sure to cool completely to prevent crumbling. For best results, wrap the cooled bread in plastic wrap or store in an airtight container for several hours or overnight before slicing. Quick breads taste and slice best when enjoyed a day after baking.

PER SERVING: 131 calories, 3 grams protein, 24 grams carbohydrates, 3 grams total fat

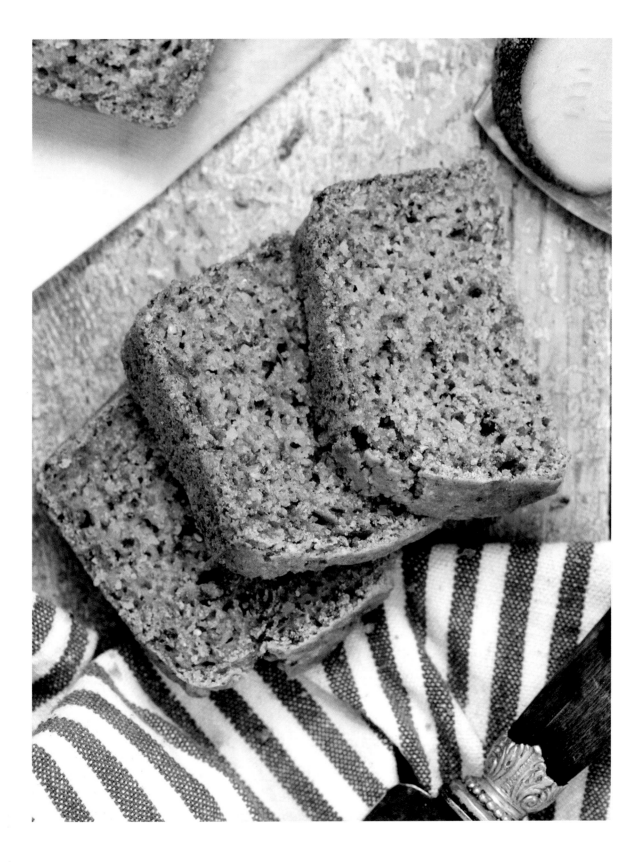

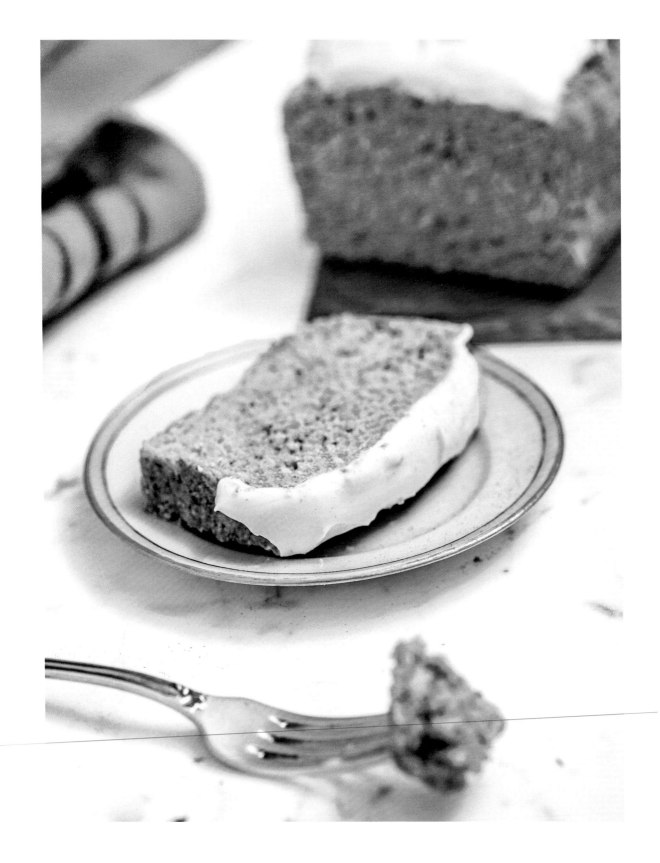

ICED PUMPKIN BREAD

▶ **NO OIL** ▶ **REFINED SUGAR-FREE**

PREP TIME: 10 min
COOK TIME: 50 min
TOTAL TIME: 60 min

MAKES ABOUT 12 SLICES

Pumpkin is great for weight loss and for heart and eye health, and it is known to help reduce the risk of cancer. This pumpkin bread is incredibly simple and easy to make, even for nonbakers.

INGREDIENTS:

¾ cup pumpkin puree

½ cup sweetened vanilla almond milk

½ cup maple syrup

2 tablespoons applesauce

1 teaspoon vanilla extract

½ teaspoon apple cider vinegar

½ cup brown rice flour

½ cup oat flour

½ cup tapioca and/or arrowroot flour

½ cup almond flour

1 tablespoon flax meal

1 tablespoon ground chia seeds

2 teaspoons baking powder

½ teaspoon baking soda

1 teaspoon ground cinnamon

¼ teaspoon nutmeg

⅛ teaspoon sea salt, optional

INGREDIENTS FOR ICING:

5 tablespoons coconut cream

3 tablespoons maple syrup

1 teaspoon vanilla extract

PREPARATION FOR ICING:

Add icing ingredients to a stand mixer bowl and whip until creamy and smooth. Set aside until ready to use.

PREPARATION:

1. Preheat oven to 350F and lightly grease a small (8" x 4") loaf pan or line it with parchment paper.

2. In a bowl, mix together the pumpkin puree, almond milk, maple syrup, applesauce, vanilla, and apple cider vinegar. Set aside.

3. In another bowl, whisk together the flours, flax meal, chia seeds, baking powder, baking soda, cinnamon, nutmeg, and salt (optional).

4. Pour the wet ingredients over the dry and stir until just combined. Do not overmix.

5. Pour the batter into the pan and bake for about 50 minutes or until a toothpick inserted in the center of the loaf comes out clean. Remove the pan from the oven and let it cool before transferring the loaf from the pan to a wire rack.

Recipe continues

6. Cool completely (about 1 or 2 hours), then coat with icing, slice, and serve! You can refrigerate the iced loaf before slicing so that the icing can slightly harden, making it easier to slice.

TIP: Leftovers can be stored in an airtight container at room temperature for no more than a few days, in the refrigerator for up to a week, or in the freezer for no more than a few months. Slices should be individually wrapped with plastic freezer wrap or layered with parchment paper in freezer bags.

NOTE: Like most quick breads, make sure to cool completely to prevent crumbling. For best results, wrap the cooled bread in plastic wrap or store in an airtight container for several hours or overnight before slicing. Quick breads taste and slice best when enjoyed a day after baking.

PER SERVING INCLUDING ICING: 180 calories, 3 grams protein, 33 grams carbohydrates, 4 grams total fat

LEMON CHIA MUFFINS

▶ **NO OIL**

PREP TIME: 10 min
COOK TIME: 24 min
TOTAL TIME: 34 min

MAKES 12 MUFFINS

Chia is the Mayan word for "strength." This might be because although these seeds are tiny, they pack a ton of nutrition. Loaded with fiber, protein, heart-healthy omega-3 fatty acids, manganese, magnesium, phosphorus, and calcium, these seeds should be a staple in every home. Here's a great way to introduce them to your family.

INGREDIENTS:

1 cup gluten-free oat flour

1 cup almond flour

½ cup organic coconut palm sugar

2 tablespoons milled chia seeds

2 tablespoons chia seeds

½ teaspoon baking soda

½ teaspoon baking powder

¾ cup sweetened vanilla almond milk

3 tablespoons applesauce

4 tablespoons lemon juice

ICING (OPTION 1):

½ cup powdered sugar

1 tablespoon lemon juice

Whisk together all ingredients.

ICING (OPTION 2):

5 tablespoons coconut cream

3 tablespoons maple syrup

1 teaspoon vanilla extract

1 tablespoon lemon juice

Whisk together all ingredients.

PREPARATION:

1. Preheat oven to 350F and lightly grease a standard 12-cup muffin pan with coconut oil or line with paper liners.

2. In a bowl, whisk together the gluten-free oat flour, almond flour, palm sugar, chia seeds, baking soda, and baking powder.

3. In another bowl, mix together the almond milk, applesauce, and lemon juice.

4. Pour the wet ingredients over the dry and stir well until consistency is smooth.

5. Pour the batter into 12 muffin tins.

6. Bake for 20 to 24 minutes or until a toothpick inserted into the center of a muffin comes out clean.

Recipe continues

7. Remove the pan from the oven and let it cool. Transfer the muffins to a wire rack to completely cool. If you desire icing, drizzle with icing before serving and enjoy!

TIP: Leftovers can be stored at room temperature in an airtight container for up to a few days, in the refrigerator for up to a week, or in the freezer, individually wrapped with freezer wrap, for up to a few months.

PER SERVING WITHOUT ICING: 162 calories, 4 grams protein, 25 grams carbohydrates, 6 grams total fat

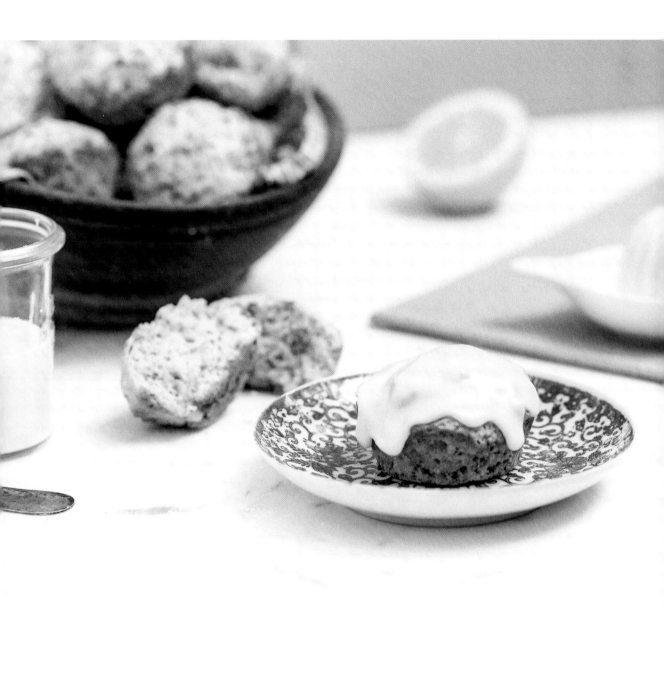

MULTIGRAIN PANCAKES WITH BERRIES & COCONUT WHIPPED CREAM

PREP TIME: 10 min

COOK TIME: 20 min

TOTAL TIME: 30 min

MAKES 8 TO 10

Indulge without the feelings that usually follow. These multigrain pancakes are full of flavor but light in calories and fat. As a bonus, we've added some protein from oats, millet, rice, and golden flax.

INGREDIENTS:

½ cup oat flour

½ cup millet flour

½ cup brown rice flour

2 tablespoons milled golden flaxseed or milled chia seeds

1½ teaspoons baking powder

¼ teaspoon baking soda

1¾ cups sweetened vanilla almond milk or other nondairy milk

2 tablespoons maple syrup

Coconut Whipped Cream (see recipe on page 324), for topping

fresh berries, for topping

maple syrup, for topping

PREPARATION:

1. In a bowl, mix the dry ingredients together. Then add the almond milk and maple syrup and stir together until well combined. Let the batter sit for a few minutes to allow it to thicken.

2. Meanwhile, lightly grease a large non-stick pan with coconut oil or another oil of your choice and heat over medium-high heat.

3. Scoop about ¼ to ½ cup of batter onto the pan for each pancake and quickly spread the batter into a circular shape, making about 4 pancakes at a time. Reduce heat to medium and let the pancakes cook for about 3 to 4 minutes, or until bubbles appear. Flip and cook the pancake for another few minutes until golden. Repeat until all batter has been used.

4. Serve and top with a scoop of Coconut Whipped Cream, fresh berries, and a drizzle of maple syrup.

TIP: Store leftovers in the freezer. When ready to enjoy, simply toast in the toaster oven until warm.

PER SERVING WITHOUT TOPPINGS: 140 calories, 3 grams protein, 25 grams carbohydrates, 3 grams total fat

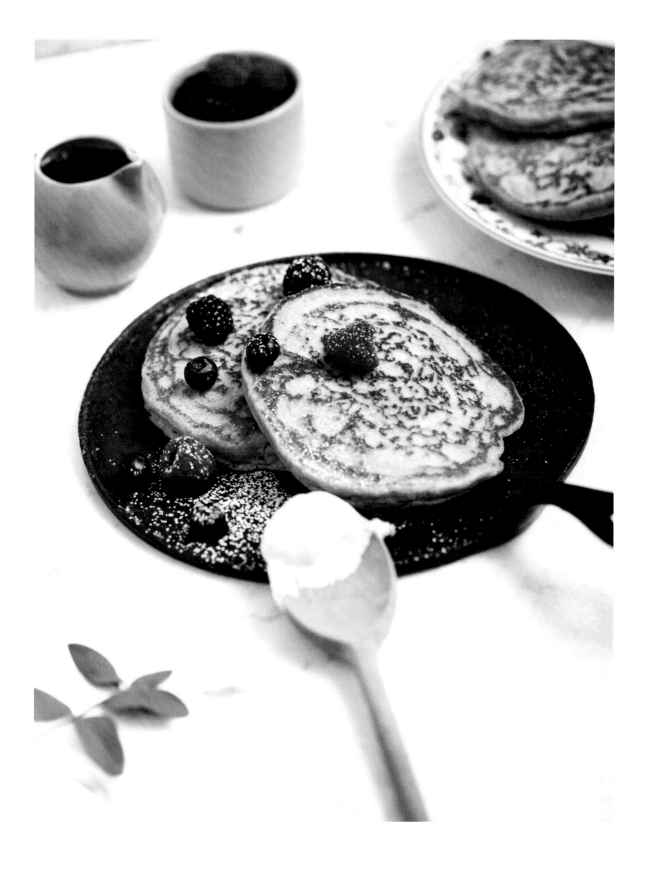

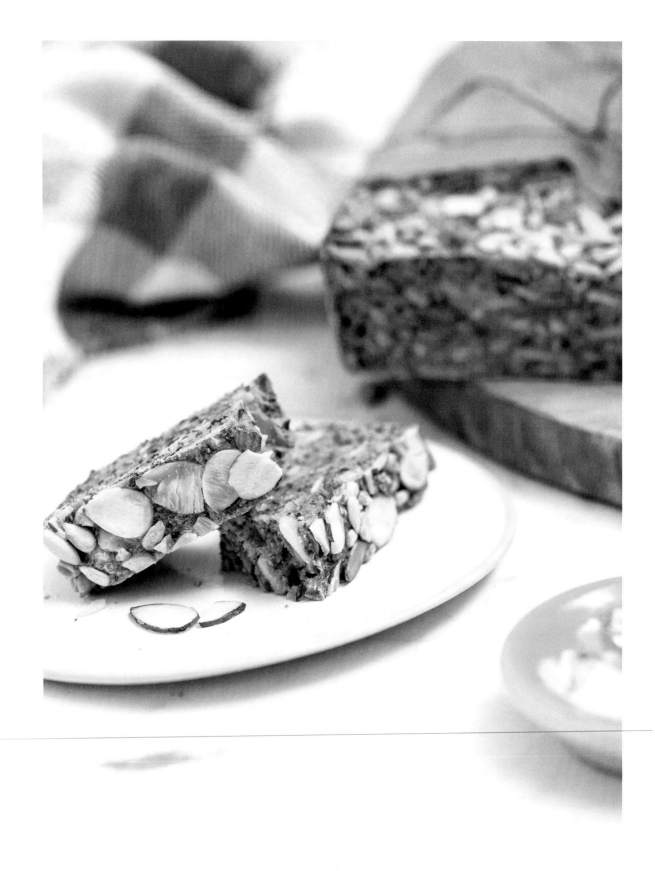

NUT AND SEED BREAD

▶ **OIL-FREE** ▶ **GRAIN-FREE OPTION**

PREP TIME: 15 min

COOK TIME: 55 min

TOTAL TIME: 70 min (doesn't include the rest time before baking)

MAKES ABOUT 18 SLICES

This hearty protein-, fiber-, and nutrient-packed bread can be enjoyed at any time of the day! It's delicious when simply toasted and/or served open-faced, topped with almond butter and fruit. It also makes a mouthwatering base for hummus and/or avocado toast—satisfying and delicious!

INGREDIENTS:

½ cup quinoa flour

½ cup gluten-free oat flour

½ cup brown rice flour

½ cup almond flour

1 cup sunflower seeds, roasted and unsalted

½ cup pumpkin seeds

½ cup almond slices

½ cup flax meal

2 tablespoons milled chia seeds

1 teaspoon sea salt

1 tablespoon psyllium husk powder

2 cups water

seeds, for sprinkling on loaf, to taste

nuts, for sprinkling on loaf, to taste

PREPARATION:

1. Line a small (8" x 4") loaf pan with parchment paper and set aside.

2. In a bowl, combine all the dry ingredients, except the psyllium husk powder, and mix well.

3. Pour the water into the dry ingredients and combine well. Mix in the psyllium husk powder, and immediately pour the thick batter into the loaf pan. Use the back of a spoon to press the batter down and smooth the top. Sprinkle the loaf with desired seeds and nuts.

4. Cover the loaf pan with a damp kitchen cloth or plastic wrap and set aside for a few hours or overnight to allow the batter to harden and the seeds to absorb the moisture.

5. When ready to cook the loaf, preheat oven to 350F and bake for 55 minutes or until the loaf is firm and lightly golden.

6. Let cool completely on a cooling rack before slicing.

Recipe continues

TIP: Store leftover bread in an airtight container at room temperature for no more than a few days, in the refrigerator for up to a week, or in the freezer for a few months. Slices should be individually wrapped with plastic freezer wrap or layered with parchment paper in freezer bags.

NOTE: To make this recipe grain-free, simply substitute 1 more cup of quinoa flour for the ½ cup oat and ½ cup brown rice flour. Also, like most quick breads, make sure to cool completely to prevent crumbling. For best results, wrap the cooled bread in plastic wrap or store in an airtight container for several hours or overnight before slicing. Quick breads taste and slice best when enjoyed a day after baking.

▶ Variation: For more variety, add ½ cup raisins, ½ cup cranberries, and ½ cup walnuts.

PER SERVING: 151 calories, 6 grams protein, 12 grams carbohydrates, 10 grams total fat

SEEDED WHOLE-GRAIN BREAD

PREP TIME: 10 min

COOK TIME: 50 min

TOTAL TIME: 60 min (does not include rising time)

MAKES ABOUT 14 SLICES

This bread is incredibly simple and delicious, and it might have you pass on commercial bread forever.

INGREDIENTS:

2 cups warm water, divided

2¼ teaspoons active dry yeast

1 teaspoon maple syrup

1 tablespoon canola oil

1½ cups oat flour

1 cup brown rice flour

½ cup quinoa flour

2 tablespoons milled chia seeds

3 tablespoons flax meal

1 teaspoon sea salt

¼ cup pumpkin seeds, set aside 1 tablespoon for topping

¼ cup sunflower seeds, set aside 1 tablespoon for topping

1 tablespoon hulled hemp seeds, for topping

1 tablespoon gluten-free oats, for topping

PREPARATION:

1. Proof the yeast: In a bowl, combine 1 cup of warm water (about 110F) with the yeast and maple syrup and allow it to froth for about 5 to 10 minutes. (The yeast mixture should get frothy and bubbly. If it doesn't, toss it out and try again.) Add the second cup of water and oil and set aside.

2. In another bowl, combine the dry ingredients, except for the pumpkin and sunflower seeds, the hemp seeds, and the gluten-free oats. Whisk well.

3. Pour the wet ingredients into the dry and stir well. Gently fold in the pumpkin and sunflower seeds.

4. Pour the batter into a small (8" x 4") loaf pan lined with parchment paper, and use the back of a spoon to gently press and smooth out the top of the batter. Sprinkle with the reserved seeds and the gluten-free oats. (Recipe image shown without seed topping.)

5. Cover the loaf pan with a damp kitchen cloth or plastic wrap and set aside to allow the loaf to rise for approximately 45 minutes. Check on the loaf after 30 minutes and remove the towel or wrap to allow the loaf to fully rise.

6. Preheat oven to 350F, then bake the loaf for about 50 minutes.

7. Remove the pan from the oven and let it cool for a few minutes before transferring the

loaf from the pan to a wire rack. Let the loaf cool completely before slicing to prevent crust from crumbling.

TIP: Store leftover bread in an airtight container at room temperature for no more than a few days, in the refrigerator for up to a week, or in the freezer for no more than a few months. Slices should be individually wrapped with plastic freezer wrap or layered with parchment paper in freezer bags.

NOTE: Plan ahead when making this bread. Allow enough time for rising and cooling prior to slicing! Also, for best results, wrap the cooled bread in plastic wrap or store in an airtight container for several hours or overnight. This bread tastes and slices best when enjoyed a day after baking.

PER SERVING: 166 calories, 6 grams protein, 23 grams carbohydrates, 6 grams total fat

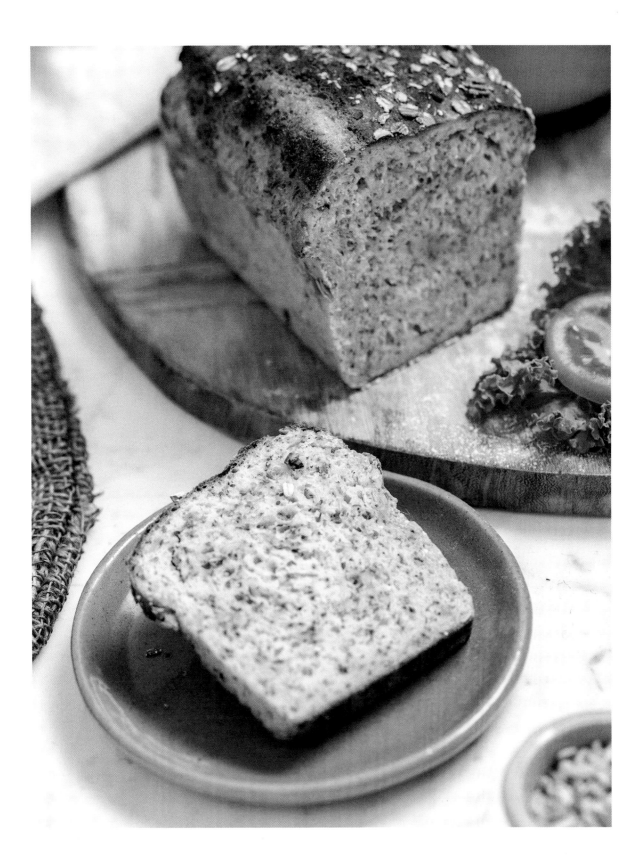

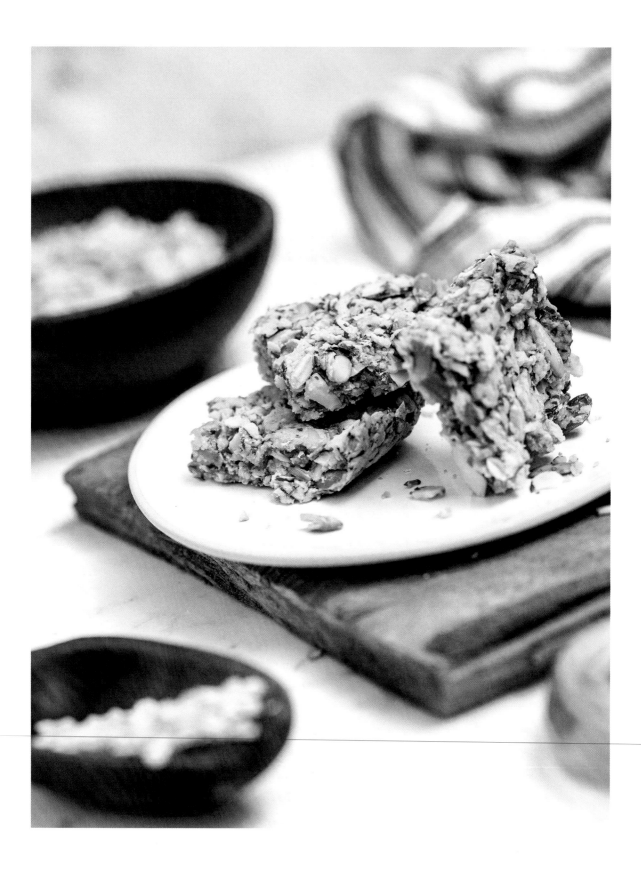

FRUIT & NUT GRANOLA BARS

PREP TIME: 20 min

COOK TIME: 25 min

TOTAL TIME: 45 min

MAKES 8 BARS

Say good-bye to commercially bought granola bars with junky ingredients. These easy-to-make granola bars are a great snack for kids, and they serve as a great pre- or intra-workout snack for adults. They're loaded with protein and fiber and are the perfect combination of crunchy and chewy.

INGREDIENTS:

¼ cup maple syrup

2 tablespoons melted coconut oil

½ cup oat flour

¼ cup instant oats

¼ cup almond meal/flour

½ cup sliced almonds

¼ cup chopped walnuts

¼ cup raisins

¼ cup pumpkin seeds

¼ cup sunflower seeds

4 tablespoons flax meal

PREPARATION:

1. Preheat oven to 350F.

2. In a bowl, mix together the maple syrup and coconut oil.

3. In another bowl, mix the remaining ingredients until well combined.

4. Stir the wet mixture into the dry and let sit for about 10 minutes so that the liquid is absorbed and the mixture thickens.

5. Thinly spread the mixture onto a parchment-lined 6" x 8" baking pan (an 8" x 8" can also work). Firmly press down, making sure the mixture is tightly packed.

6. Transfer the pan to the freezer for about 10 minutes to allow the mixture to firm up, making it easier to cut without crumbling.

7. Remove the pan from the freezer and carefully cut the mixture into 8 rectangular shapes using a pastry scraper or knife.

8. Bake for 20 to 25 minutes.

9. Place the pan on a cooling rack for about 15 minutes. Then carefully separate the mixture into individual bars and transfer them back to the cooling rack.

10. Let the bars cool completely for a crunchier texture.

TIP: Store leftovers in an airtight container, individually wrapped or layered with parchment paper, at room temperature for no more than a few days, in the refrigerator for up to a week, or in the freezer for no more than a month.

PER SERVING: 371 calories, 11 grams protein, 27 grams carbohydrates, 28 grams total fat

GRANOLA

PREP TIME: 5 min

COOK TIME: 20 min

TOTAL TIME: 25 min

MAKES 6 SERVINGS (⅔ CUP EACH)

Who doesn't love crunchy sweetness for breakfast? Well, this time, we get it, without the guilt that usually comes with it. This homemade crispy mix of oats, nuts, and seeds will be sure to satisfy even the most seasoned sweet tooth.

INGREDIENTS:

2 cups quick oats

1½ cups rolled oats

½ cup maple syrup

2 tablespoons pumpkin seeds

2 tablespoons sliced almonds

2 tablespoons cashews, chopped

1 tablespoon milled flaxseed

¼ teaspoon ground cinnamon

PREPARATION:

1. Preheat oven to 350F.

2. In a large mixing bowl, toss together all ingredients.

3. Place granola mixture on a baking sheet lined with parchment paper and bake for 18 to 20 minutes until golden brown, tossing once halfway through cooking time.

4. Remove from the oven and let cool completely.

TIP: To serve, pour about ⅔ of a cup of granola into a bowl with ½ cup of almond milk, and enjoy! Feel free to top with fresh fruit of choice. Store in an airtight container until ready to use. Leftovers can be stored at room temperature for up to 1 week or in the refrigerator for up to 1 month.

VARIATION

▸ Granola Clusters (makes 6 servings): Process 1 cup of the rolled oats into flour, and add 1 tablespoon of melted coconut oil to the mixture above. Then firmly press the mixture down onto the baking sheet, and follow the same cooking instructions, except you will need to break up the granola into clusters once it's done baking and completely cooled. Follow the same serving suggestions as above.

PER SERVING: 301 calories, 8 grams protein, 52 grams carbohydrates, 7 grams total fat

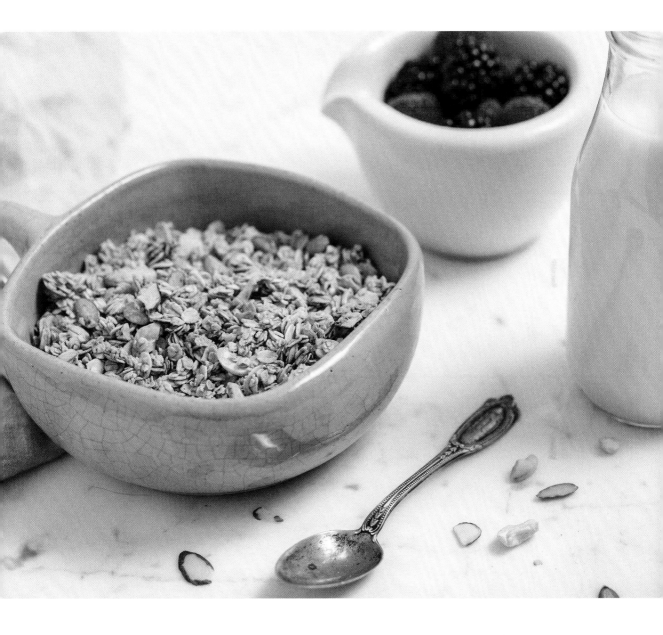

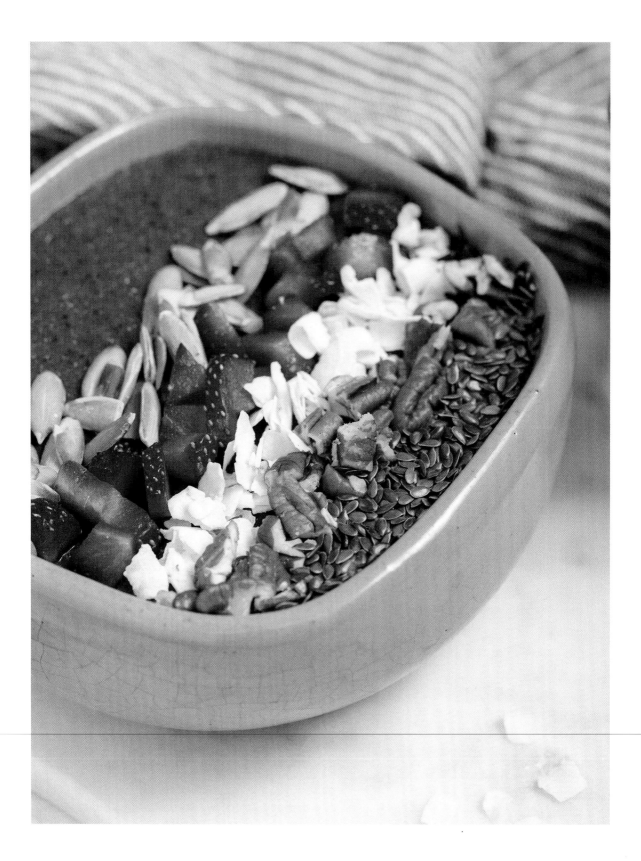

ACAI POWER BOWL

PREP TIME: 15 min

COOK TIME: 10 min

TOTAL TIME: 25 min

MAKES 2 SERVINGS

This breakfast bowl is packed with powerful antioxidants (found in kale, acai, blueberries, and chia). They contain key phytochemicals known to protect against cancer and heart disease, as well as vitamins and minerals that help strengthen the immune system.

Blueberries, in particular, may help lower inflammation and protect cells from damage, and superstar dark green veggies, such as kale or spinach, are high in magnesium, manganese, potassium, and calcium, as well as vitamins K, C, E and A. Acai, sourced in the Brazilian Amazon, also contains heart-healthy omega-3 fatty acids. And chia seeds are not only rich in omega-3s, but also in fiber and protein. Real energy from real food!

INGREDIENTS:

½ cup chopped kale, without stalks

½ cup frozen blueberries

1 frozen banana

2 teaspoons milled chia seeds or milled flaxseed

1 scoop 22 Days Plant-Protein Powder

1 cup sweetened vanilla almond milk or other nondairy beverage of choice

1 3.5-ounce acai smoothie pack, frozen and unsweetened

OPTIONAL TOPPINGS:

Granola (see recipe on page 60)

fruit

nuts

seeds (such as hemp, chia, or flax)

PREPARATION:

1. Prepare the toppings of your choice and set them aside until ready to use.

2. For the acai smoothie, place ingredients into a blender in this order: kale, blueberries, banana, chia or flax meal, 22 Days Plant Protein, almond milk, and acai. (Thaw the frozen acai pulp by running under water for a few seconds, then open the pack and break the contents into pieces. Placing unfrozen ingredients in the blender first makes it easier to blend them together.)

3. Blend the ingredients until smooth, stopping to scrape down the sides if necessary.

4. Pour the acai smoothie into two bowls and finish with the toppings of choice.

PER SERVING WITHOUT OPTIONAL TOPPINGS:
249 calories, 11 grams protein, 41 grams carbohydrates, 6 grams total fat

BERRY VANILLA CHIA PUDDING

PREP TIME: 5 min

COOK TIME: 0 min

TOTAL TIME: 5 min (does not include overnight refrigeration)

MAKES 2 SERVINGS

We love the taste of this pudding! It might take a few tries before you get used to the taste and texture of chia, but the nutritional benefits are more than worth the few extra tries. Chia is loaded with heart-healthy omega-3 fatty acids, fiber, protein, manganese, magnesium, and phosphorus, which make for an amazing start to any day.

INGREDIENTS:

½ cup chia seeds

2 cups sweetened vanilla almond milk or non-dairy beverage of choice

1 teaspoon vanilla extract

2 tablespoons maple syrup

1 cup berries

PREPARATION:

1. Stir together all ingredients in a bowl until well combined.

2. Store the pudding in an airtight glass container (with a lid) in the refrigerator overnight.

3. When ready to serve, stir pudding well and spoon into a bowl. Top with berries and enjoy!

PER SERVING: 309 calories, 8 grams protein, 50 grams carbohydrates, 12 grams total fat

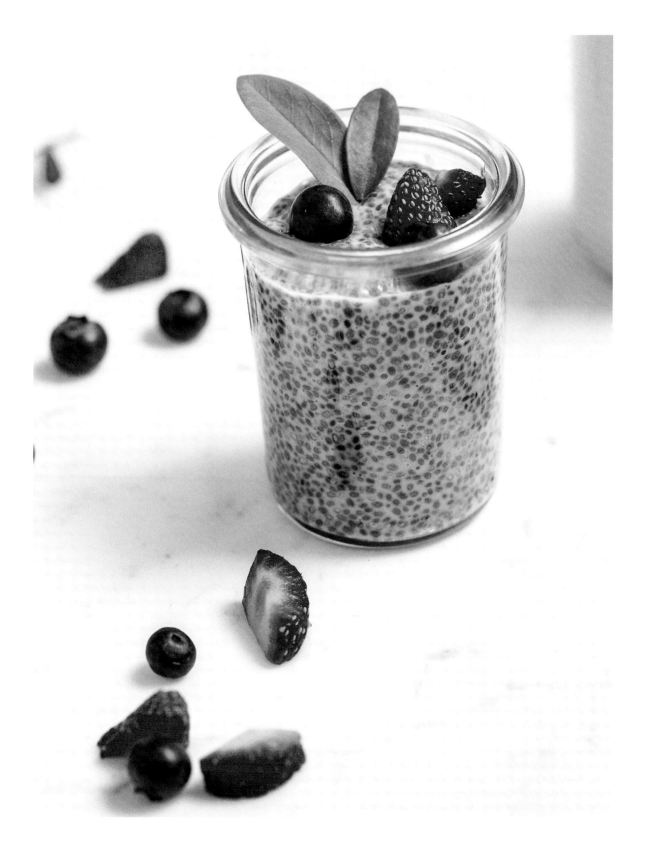

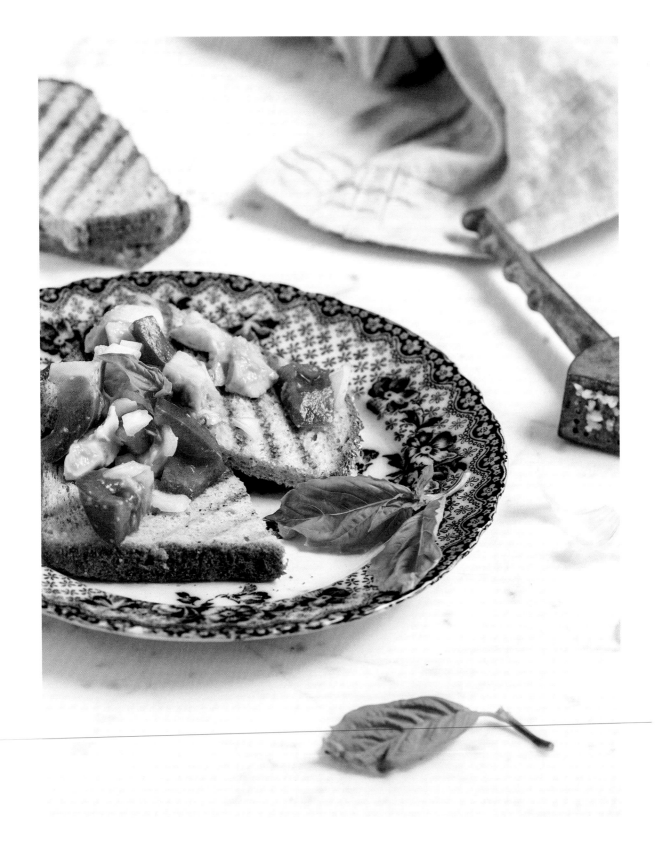

AVOCADO TOMATO BRUSCHETTA

PREP TIME: 10 min

COOK TIME: 5 min

TOTAL TIME: 15 min

MAKES 2 SERVINGS

This recipe is delicious with the Seeded Whole-Grain Bread (see recipe on page 55) or the Nut and Seed Bread (see recipe on page 53). It can be enjoyed for breakfast or as an appetizer.

INGREDIENTS:

1 Hass avocado, halved, pitted, peeled, and diced

1 medium tomato, finely chopped

¼ small onion, diced

1 garlic clove, minced

3 tablespoons lemon juice

2 teaspoons extra-virgin olive oil

1 tablespoon balsamic vinegar

pinch of dried basil flakes

sea salt, to taste

ground black pepper, to taste

3 slices gluten-free bread

PREPARATION:

1. In a mixing bowl, toss all ingredients together, except the bread.

2. Toast the bread, slice in halves, top with the avocado mixture, and serve!

PER SERVING: 317 calories, 4 grams protein, 38 grams carbohydrates, 18 grams total fat

POTATO LATKES

PREP TIME: 15 min

COOK TIME: 20 min

TOTAL TIME: 35 min

MAKES 4 SERVINGS

Hot and crunchy . . . sign me up! Unfairly cast aside because of low-carb diets due to their starchy makeup, potatoes have fallen off our menus. Here are a few good reasons to consider bringing them back. Potatoes are low in calories and fat but are loaded with vitamin C, vitamin B$_6$, calcium, potassium, protein, and fiber. Additionally, potatoes contain a compound known as ALA (alpha-lipoic acid), which helps the body convert glucose into energy.

INGREDIENTS:

2 large russet potatoes (about 1½ to 2 pounds), washed, peeled, and grated

1 small onion, grated

¼ cup quinoa flour or oat flour

1 teaspoon baking powder

1 tablespoon milled chia seeds

1 teaspoon sea salt, or to taste

ground black pepper, to taste

4 tablespoons canola oil, for cooking

parsley flakes, for garnish

PREPARATION:

1. Place grated potatoes in a bowl of water to stop them from turning brown while you assemble your ingredients.

2. Rinse the grated potatoes in a large colander until the water comes out clear. This step helps remove the starch and makes it easier to get a crispy latke. Squeeze out the excess water.

3. In a bowl, mix the potatoes with the onion, flour, baking powder, milled chia seeds, salt, and pepper.

4. Heat 1 to 2 tablespoons of oil in a large nonstick pan over medium-high heat.

5. Reduce heat to medium and scoop out ½ cup of the potato mixture, per latke, into the skillet. Lightly flatten the potato latke with a spatula, making 4 small latkes at a time.

6. Cook for 4 to 5 minutes per side, until golden brown and crispy. Make the rest of the latkes, adding 1 to 2 tablespoons of oil to the pan for cooking, until all the batter has been used. Should make about 8 latkes as an appetizer, and 4 as an entrée.

7. Place the latkes on a plate lined with a paper towel, to drain. Serve and garnish with chopped parsley.

PER SERVING: 305 calories, 5 grams protein, 40 grams carbohydrates, 15 grams total fat

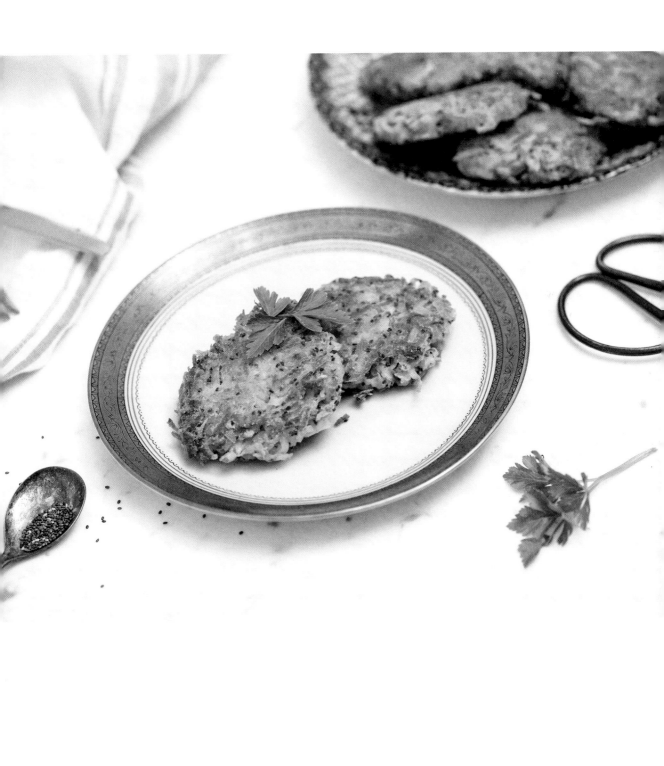

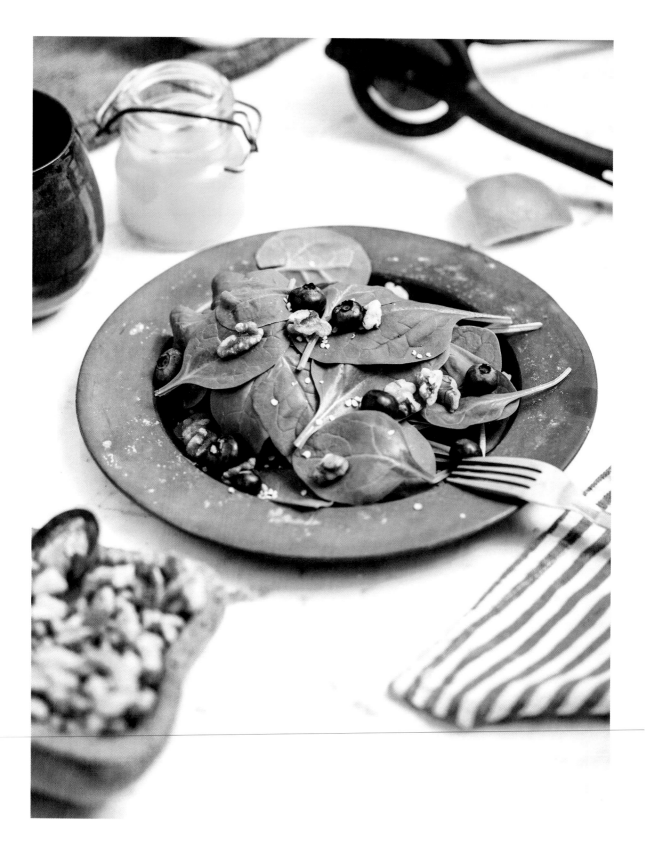

SPINACH AND BERRIES BREAKFAST SALAD

PREP TIME: 10 min

COOK TIME: 0 min

TOTAL TIME: 10 min

MAKES 1 SERVING

This recipe flips or rather tosses the idea of breakfast on its head. Spinach is known for many health benefits, including healthy skin and hair, cancer prevention, lowering blood pressure, and promoting regularity. It's loaded with vitamin K, vitamin A, manganese, folate, magnesium, iron, B vitamins, calcium, vitamin C, fiber, potassium—and it doesn't end there. This light and delicious breakfast salad is exactly what the doctor ordered.

INGREDIENTS:

2 cups fresh spinach

1 cup fresh berries (an even blend of blackberries, raspberries, blueberries, and strawberries)

¼ cup chopped walnuts

1 tablespoon hulled hemp seeds

4 tablespoons fresh squeezed orange juice

PREPARATION:

1. Place a bed of spinach on a plate and top neatly with the fresh berries.

2. Sprinkle the spinach and berries with chopped walnuts and hulled hemp seeds.

3. Dress the salad with fresh orange juice.

PER SERVING: 340 calories, 11 grams protein, 27 grams carbohydrates, 25 grams total fat

BERRY MANGO HEMP SMOOTHIE

PREP TIME: 5 min

COOK TIME: 0 min

TOTAL TIME: 5 min

MAKES 1 SERVING

Kids love sugary juices and smoothies, but unfortunately the love is never reciprocated. But this love is no longer unrequited because this smoothie is full of vitamins, minerals, protein, and flavor. It's quick, easy, and good at any time of the day.

INGREDIENTS:

1 cup frozen mango chunks

2 tablespoons hulled hemp seeds, with some set aside for garnish

1 cup coconut milk or other nondairy milk of choice

1 cup frozen mixed berries

PREPARATION:

1. In a blender, blend all the ingredients together (minus a pinch of hemp seeds) until smooth.

2. Evenly pour the smoothie into 2 glasses.

3. Sprinkle each glass with the remaining hemp seeds and enjoy!

PER SERVING: 382 calories, 10 grams protein, 62 grams carbohydrates, 15 grams total fat

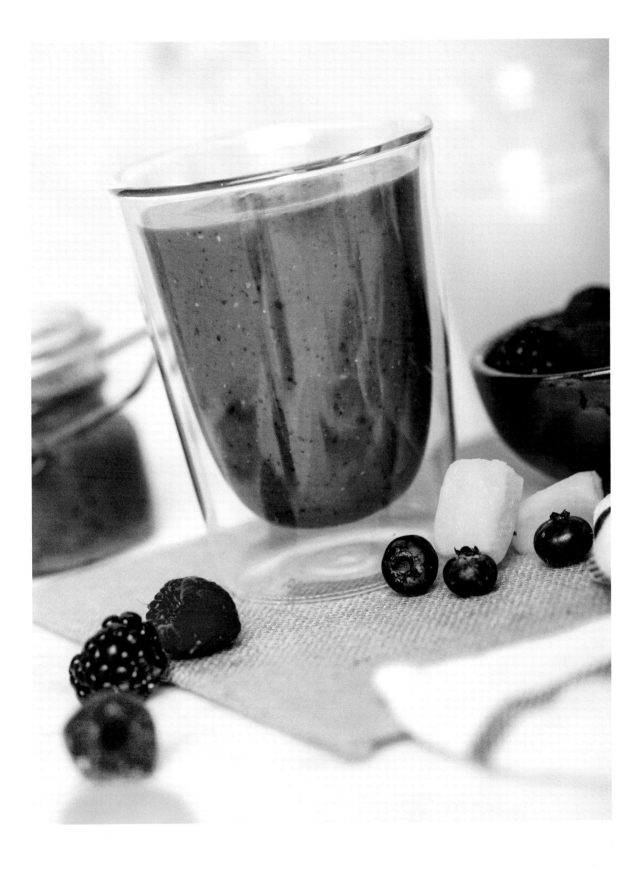

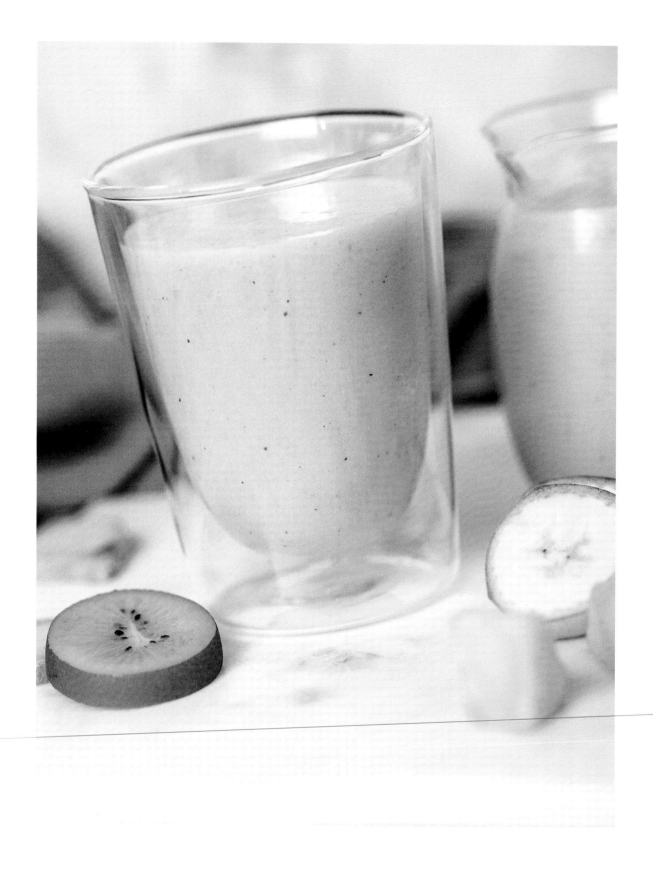

IMMUNITY-BOOSTING TROPICAL SMOOTHIE

PREP TIME: 5 min
COOK TIME: 0 min
TOTAL TIME: 5 min

MAKES 1 SERVING

This smoothie is packed with antioxidants and superfoods to uplift and recharge.

Ginger: Known for its anti-inflammatory properties, but did you know it also helps reduce nausea and pain, relieves upset stomachs, stimulates circulation, and may help prevent stomach ulcers? It's always my first choice to use fresh ginger in recipes, but keeping some prepped in the freezer can be extremely convenient. (It keeps for up to a few months.) Simply peel the ginger, cut it into ¼- to ½-inch pieces, and store it in an airtight container. Another option is to simply use ground ginger.

Turmeric: Curcumin is the active ingredient in turmeric, which is antiviral and antifungal and helps protect against cancer. Among many foods, it's known to have some of the highest antioxidant and anti-inflammatory properties.

Black pepper: This smoothie also includes black pepper, which helps increase the body's absorption significantly.

Probiotics: These boost the immune system, aid in digestion, and are ideal for maintaining a healthy gut.

Pineapple: An antioxidant-rich powerhouse with many unique health-promoting compounds, vitamins, and minerals essential for optimum health.

Kiwi: This fruit is high in fiber, and it contains more vitamin C than an orange.

INGREDIENTS:

1 cup orange juice, freshly squeezed

1 frozen banana

1 kiwi, peeled

½ cup frozen pineapple chunks

1 teaspoon probiotics powder (nondairy)

¼-inch piece fresh turmeric or ¼ teaspoon ground

¼-inch piece fresh ginger, peeled, or ¼ teaspoon ground

¼ teaspoon ground black pepper

1 large scoop ice

PREPARATION:

Combine all the ingredients in a blender and blend until smooth. Enjoy immediately to get the best of the nutritional benefits.

PER SERVING: 313 calories, 5 grams protein, 77 grams carbohydrates, 2 grams total fat

STRAWBERRY PROTEIN SMOOTHIE

PREP TIME: 5 min

COOK TIME: 0 min

TOTAL TIME: 5 min

MAKES 1 SERVING

When I was a kid, I used to spend a lot of time at my grandmother Mima's house. Like clockwork, every afternoon an ice-cream truck would drive by, and the sound of the jingle it played over a loudspeaker would have all the neighborhood kids chasing it down the street. We didn't always have the fifty cents for my favorite ice cream, but when we did, it was almost always a strawberry shortcake bar. Here's my version of it, in a smoothie.

INGREDIENTS:

1 cup frozen strawberries

1 frozen banana

1 cup almond milk or other nondairy milk of choice

1 scoop 22 Days Plant-Protein Powder

PREPARATION:

1. Blend all ingredients together in a blender until smooth.

2. Serve and enjoy!

PER SERVING: 177 calories, 10 grams protein, 30 grams carbohydrates, 3 grams total fat

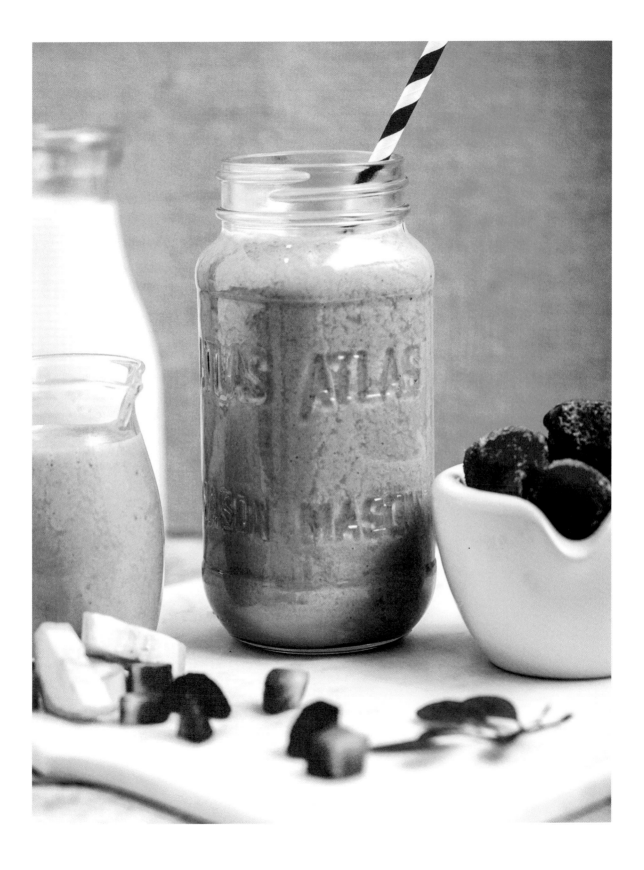

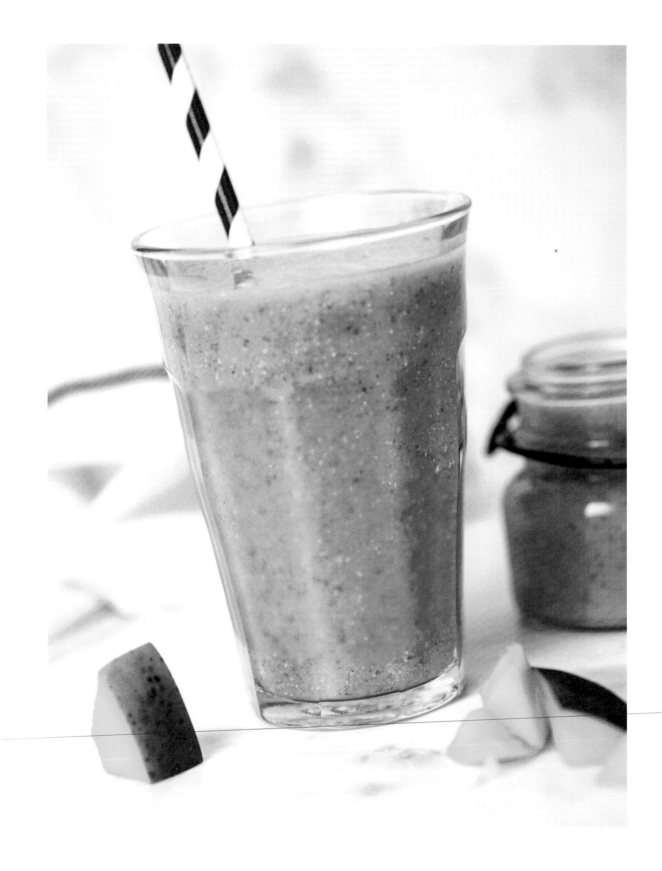

EASY DIGEST

PREP TIME: 5 min
COOK TIME: 0 min
TOTAL TIME: 5 min

MAKES 1 SERVING

Papaya is a wonderful digestive aid that contains an enzyme known as papain, which helps improve digestive health. Probiotics, chia seeds, and mango form the perfect digestive assist.

INGREDIENTS:

1 cup frozen papaya chunks

1 cup frozen mango chunks

1 tablespoon milled chia seeds

1 teaspoon probiotics

PREPARATION:

1. Blend all ingredients together in a blender until smooth.

2. Serve and enjoy!

PER SERVING: 233 calories, 4 grams protein, 53 grams carbohydrates, 3 grams total fat

GREEN DETOX JUICE

PREP TIME: 10 min

COOK TIME: 0 min

TOTAL TIME: 10 min

MAKES 1 SERVING

This juice is a good source of iron, calcium, and antioxidants, as well as vitamins A, B, C and K. This helps boost your immune system and detoxify your liver, while keeping you hydrated and energized.

INGREDIENTS:

5 stalks kale

3 green apples

1 cucumber

1 celery stalk

1 lemon, peeled

½-inch piece ginger

PREPARATION:

Juice all ingredients in a juicer, and enjoy!

PER SERVING: 388 calories, 7 grams protein, 99 grams carbohydrates, 2 gram total fat

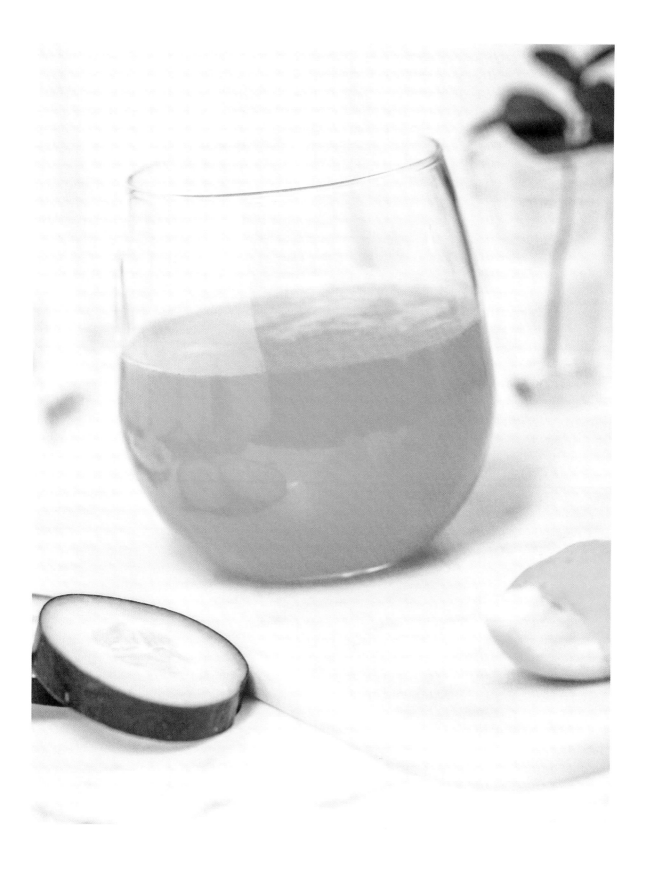

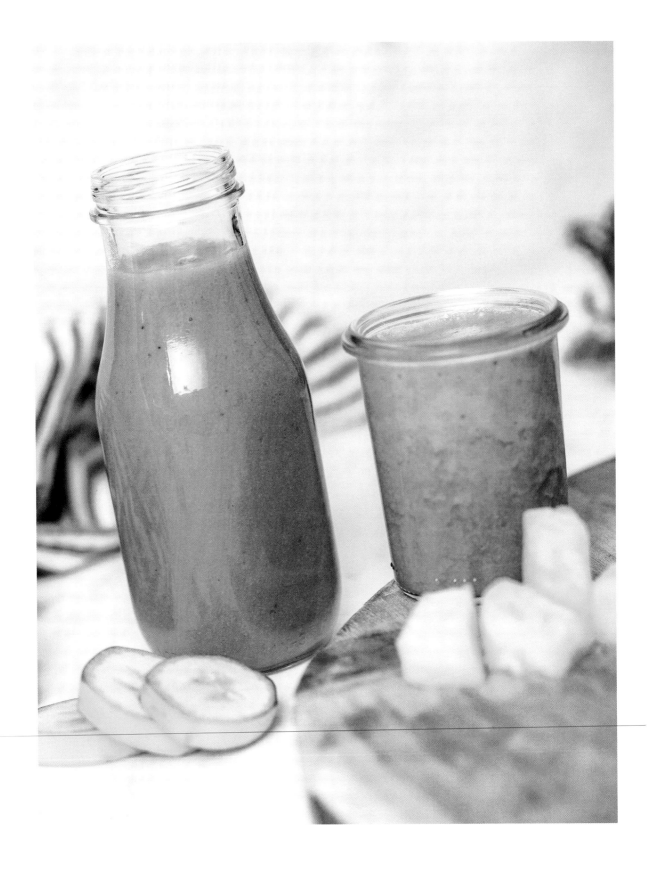

METABOLISM KICK

PREP TIME: 5 min

COOK TIME: 0 min

TOTAL TIME: 5 min

MAKES 1 SERVING

A powerhouse of nutrition, with vitamins A and C, fiber, calcium, and protein, this smoothie helps detoxify and rejuvenate the body.

INGREDIENTS:

1 frozen banana

1 cup pineapple

1 cup kale

½ cup coconut water

1 scoop 22 Days Plant-Protein Powder

PREPARATION:

1. Blend all ingredients together in a blender until smooth.

2. Serve and enjoy!

PER SERVING: 337 calories, 21 grams protein, 62 grams carbohydrates, 4 grams total fat

PROTEIN PUNCH

PREP TIME: 5 min

COOK TIME: 0 min

TOTAL TIME: 5 min

MAKES 1 SERVING

Spirulina is a natural algae that's rich in protein and high in iron and omega-3 fatty acids, and it contains more calcium than regular cow's milk.

INGREDIENTS:

1 frozen banana

1 cup frozen blackberries or blueberries

1 cup kale

1 cup spinach

1 lemon, juiced

1 cup coconut water

1 teaspoon spirulina

1 scoop vanilla 22 Days Plant-Protein Powder

PREPARATION:

1. Blend all ingredients together in a blender until smooth.

2. Serve and enjoy!

PER SERVING: 365 calories, 23 grams protein, 67 grams carbohydrates, 4 grams total fat

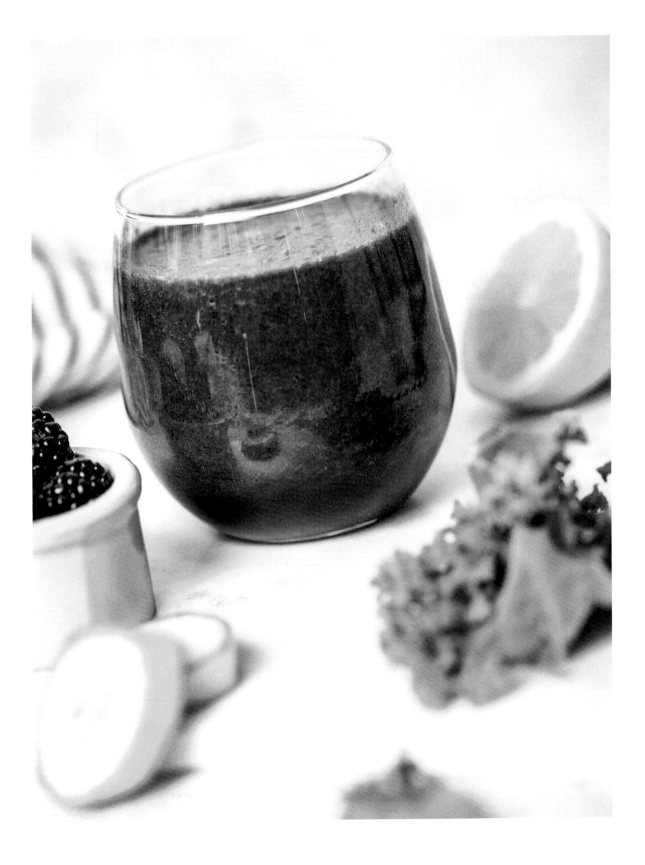

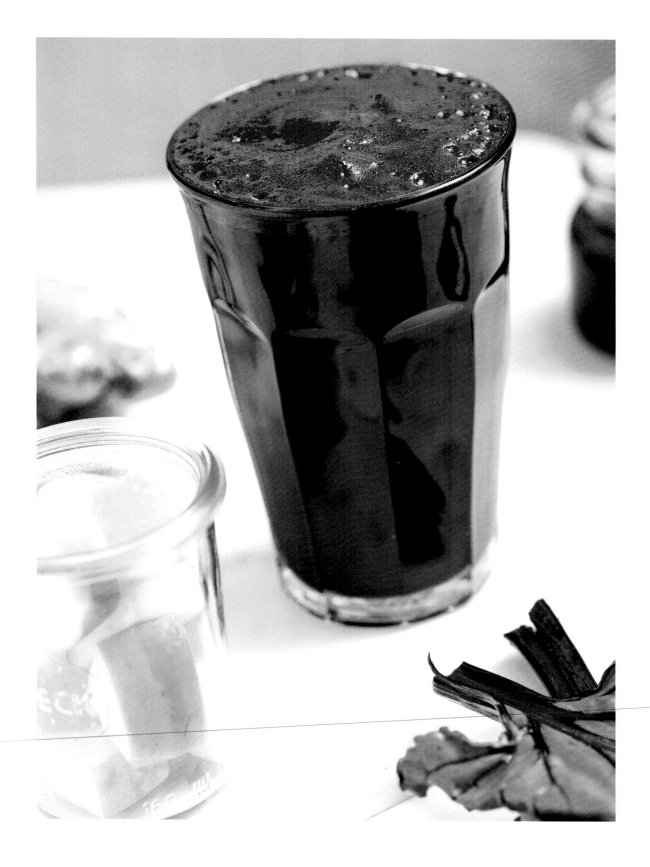

RADIANT BEET JUICE

PREP TIME: 10 min

COOK TIME: 0 min

TOTAL TIME: 10 min

MAKES 1 SERVING

Beets are highly nutritious, and they supply significant amounts of folate, manganese, copper, phosphorus, zinc, vitamins A, B_6, and C, potassium, calcium, iron, fiber, and protein. More reasons to include beets in your diet: They boost stamina, fight inflammation, improve circulation, cure anemia, calm the nerves, lower blood pressure, help detoxify, and have anticancer properties.

INGREDIENTS:

2 small beets

2 carrots

1 orange, peeled

½-inch piece turmeric

½-inch piece ginger

PREPARATION:

Juice all ingredients in a juicer, and enjoy!

PER SERVING: 169 calories, 5 grams protein, 39 grams carbohydrates, 1 gram total fat

REBOOT JUICE

PREP TIME: 10 min

COOK TIME: 0 min

TOTAL TIME: 10 min

MAKES 2 SERVINGS

Papaya is known to reduce the risk of heart disease, diabetes, and cancer, as well as lower cholesterol, boost immunity, improve digestion, protect against arthritis, and help lower blood pressure, and it is great for reducing stress.

INGREDIENTS:

1 small pineapple, peeled, cored, and sliced

1 ripe papaya, peeled, seeded, and sliced

1 ruby grapefruit, peeled

1 lemon, peeled

½-inch piece ginger

PREPARATION:

Juice all ingredients in a juicer, and enjoy!

PER SERVING: 326 calories, 4 grams protein, 85 grams carbohydrates, 1 gram total fat

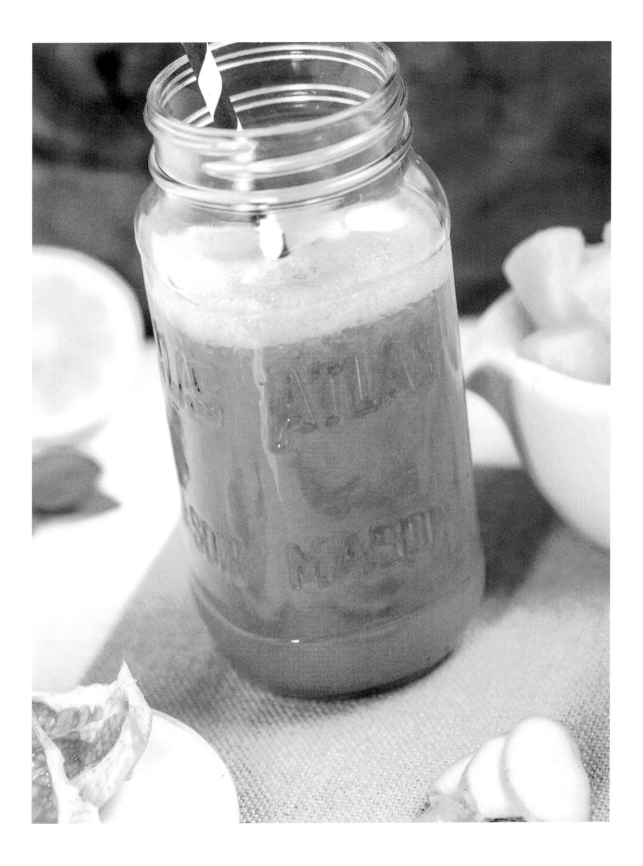

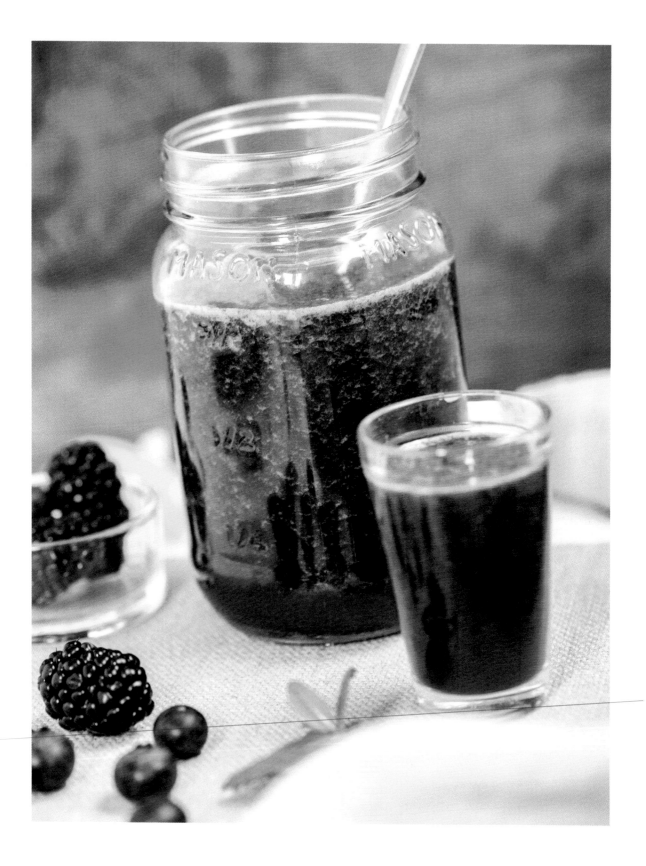

REJUVENATE JUICE

PREP TIME: 10 min

COOK TIME: 0 min

TOTAL TIME: 10 min

MAKES 1 SERVING

This juice is a powerhouse for rejuvenation and vibrant skin.

Blueberries and blackberries are full of polyphenol antioxidants, which fight free radicals and regulate the skin's blood flow, giving off a youthful glow. Mint refreshes and rejuvenates the skin and contains salicylic acid, which is a natural acne-fighting compound. Watercress not only nourishes the skin, but it is also a powerful cleansing agent that helps flush out toxins and excess fluids. Cucumber is a natural diuretic with cooling properties that can reduce redness and inflammation. Lemon is a superstar for many reasons, especially for being a natural digestive and liver cleanser.

INGREDIENTS:

1 cup blackberries

1 cup blueberries

1 cup watercress

1 small cucumber

4 mint leaves

1 lemon, peeled

PREPARATION:

Juice all ingredients in a juicer, and enjoy!

PER SERVING: 184 calories, 5 grams protein, 44 grams carbohydrates, 2 grams total fat

COCONUT YOGURT PARFAIT

PREP TIME: 20 min

COOK TIME: 20 min

TOTAL TIME: 40 min (includes Granola recipe, but doesn't include coconut milk overnight refrigeration)

MAKES 3 SERVINGS

This is as beautiful as it is healthy, and it makes any morning feel decadent while still nourishing the body.

INGREDIENTS FOR RASPBERRY JAM:

¾ cup raspberries

1 tablespoon maple syrup

INGREDIENTS FOR COCONUT YOGURT:

1 can full-fat coconut milk

¼ cup coconut water (set aside from cans; see preparation instructions)

1 teaspoon probiotic powder

1 tablespoon maple syrup or to taste

1 teaspoon vanilla extract

INGREDIENTS FOR PARFAIT:

coconut yogurt

1 cup Granola (see recipe on page 60)

¼ cup raspberries

PREPARATION:

1. Prepare the raspberry jam: In a bowl, smash the raspberries with a fork and mix together with the maple syrup.

2. Prepare the coconut yogurt: Refrigerate the can of coconut milk overnight. Then remove the can from the refrigerator and open it to scoop out the solid coconut cream, while setting aside ¼ cup of the coconut water. Transfer the coconut cream into a mixing bowl, together with probiotic powder and maple syrup and beat the cream using an electric hand mixer or stand mixer, until smooth and creamy. Continue to beat while adding the coconut water 1 tablespoon at a time until desired consistency is reached. The coconut yogurt will slightly harden as it chills.

3. Store yogurt in the refrigerator in an airtight glass container until ready to use. Can be premade and kept in the refrigerator for 2–3 days.

4. To assemble each parfait, layer 3 serving cups or small jars with even amounts of coconut yogurt, granola, and raspberry jam, repeating one more layer of coconut yogurt, granola, and raspberries.

PER SERVING: 354 calories, 5 grams protein, 34 grams carbohydrates, 24 grams total fat

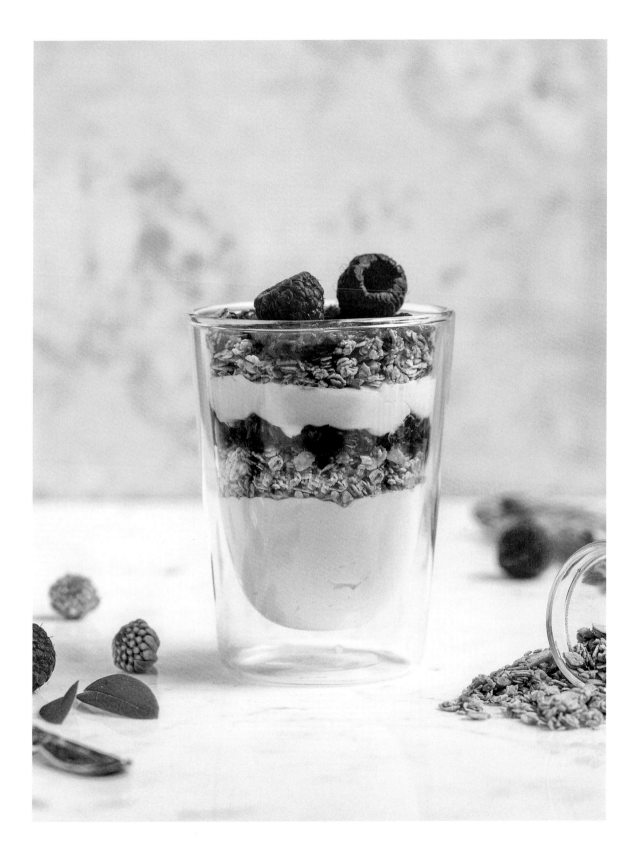

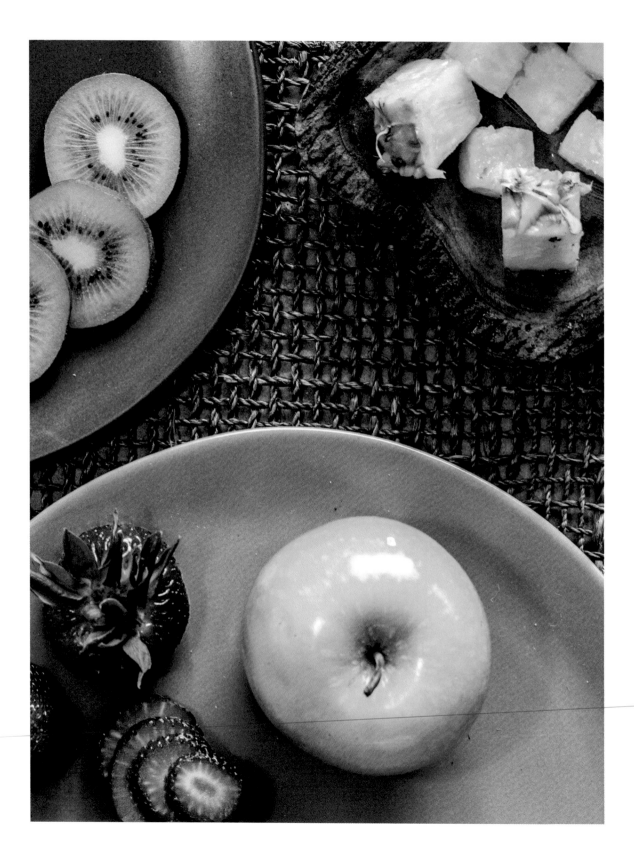

INDULGENT BREAKFASTS

(400 OR MORE CALORIES)

My wife and I are early risers and love mornings. We passed on that appreciation to our kids! You can catch us having dance-offs or going for runs, bike rides, and even walks before school. Breakfast is definitely a favorite meal for us all to fuel up for some of our family activities. These breakfast meals are intended to set the tone for the day—a tone of optimum health.

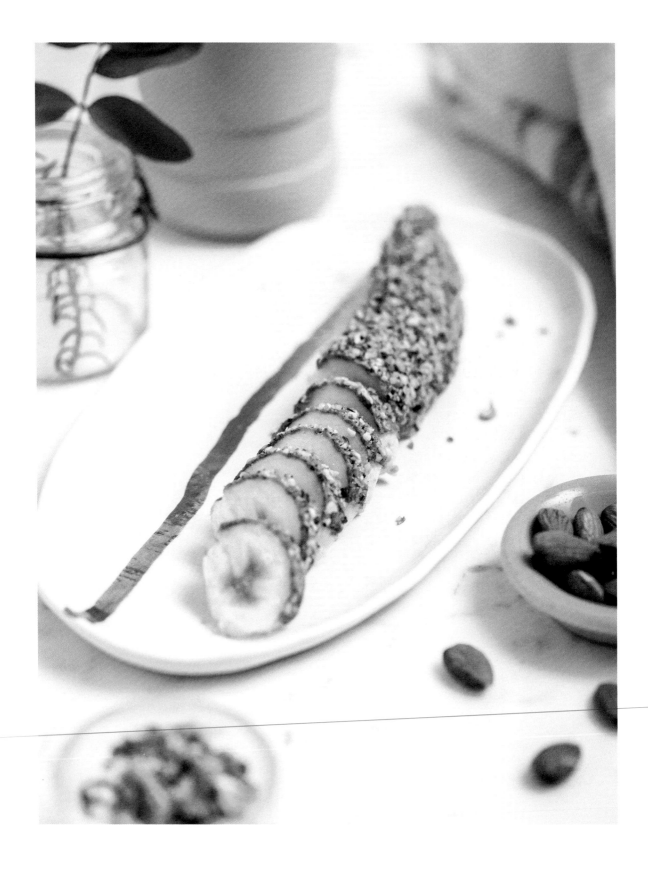

BANANA SUSHI

PREP TIME: 10 min

COOK TIME: 0 min

TOTAL TIME: 10 min (doesn't include freezer time)

MAKES 1 SERVING

Yes, banana and sushi do have something in common. This idea came to me as I was coming up with creative ways to serve my boys breakfast before school. Bananas are loaded with tryptophan, which is converted in the brain into serotonin (a happy-mood neurotransmitter), and potassium, which protects against muscle cramps during exercise. What better way to arm your kids (or yourself) for a day of happiness and health?

INGREDIENTS:

1 large banana

2 tablespoons almond butter or sunflower butter

2 tablespoons hulled hemp seeds or sesame seeds

2 tablespoons chopped pistachios

PREPARATION:

1. Peel the banana and place on parchment paper.

2. Spread butter evenly to cover just the top half of the banana, lengthwise.

3. Spread and press the hemp seeds and pistachios over the coated half.

4. Slice the banana evenly and place it in the freezer for a couple of hours.

TIP: If not consuming the banana sushi the same day you make it, you may want to transfer it to a storage container to avoid the parchment paper sticking to the coated banana.

PER SERVING: 506 calories, 18 grams protein, 45 grams carbohydrates, 34 grams total fat

CHOCOLATE BANANA PROTEIN PUDDING

PREP TIME: 10 min

COOK TIME: 0 min

TOTAL TIME: 10 min

MAKES 1 SERVING

If you love working out before breakfast, you'll love this. It's the perfect post-workout recovery smoothie-turned-pudding! Chocolate and protein. What more can an athlete ask for? And for an extra touch of richness, top with a scoop of Coconut Whipped Cream (see recipe on page 324).

INGREDIENTS:

½ cup sweetened vanilla almond milk or other nondairy beverage of choice

1 frozen banana

1 tablespoon maple syrup

1 tablespoon cocoa powder, plus extra for dusting

1 tablespoon almond butter or nut butter of choice

1 scoop 22 Days Plant-Protein Powder

sliced strawberries, for topping

PREPARATION:

1. Add all ingredients except the strawberries to a blender or food processor and process, stopping to scrape down the sides, until pudding reaches a smooth and creamy consistency.

2. Serve and top with fresh strawberries and a dusting of cocoa powder!

PER SERVING: 436 calories, 22 grams protein, 61 grams carbohydrates, 13 grams total fat

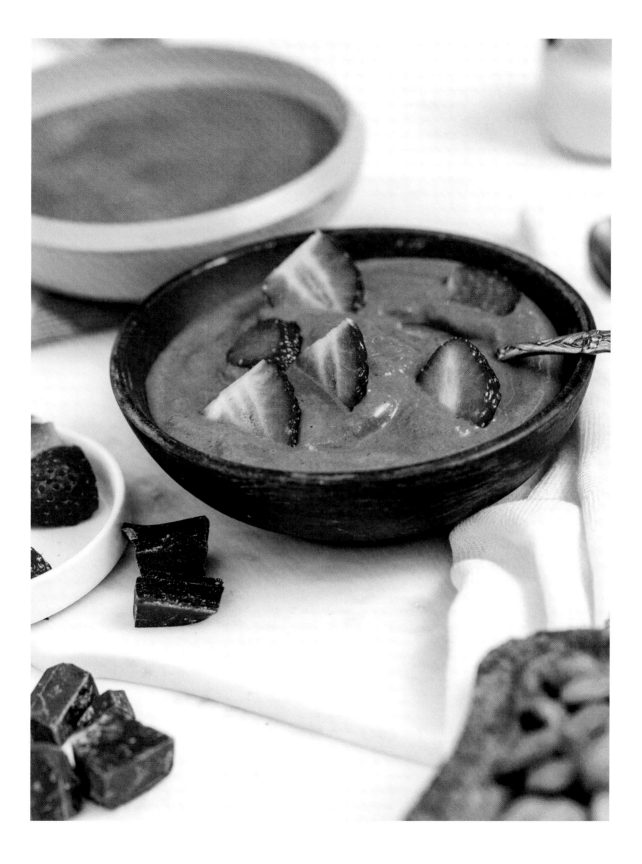

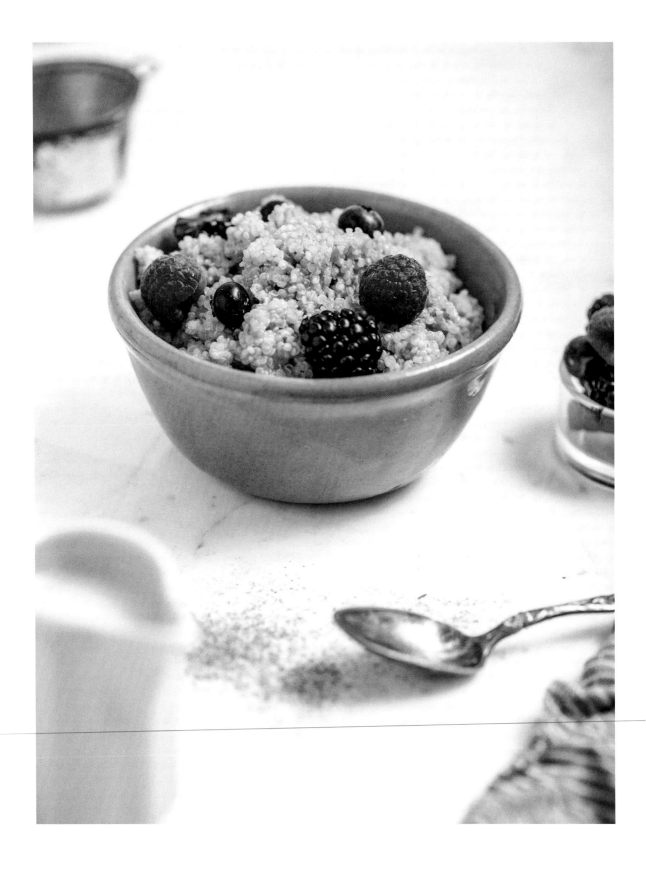

BREAKFAST QUINOA

PREP TIME: 5 min

COOK TIME: 20 min

TOTAL TIME: 25 min

MAKES 2 SERVINGS

Quinoa is an ancient seed known for being one of only a few plants considered a complete protein (which means it contains all essential amino acids), making it a perfect food. This hearty breakfast is loaded with antioxidants and protein for a perfect start to any morning.

INGREDIENTS:

1 cup quinoa

¾ cup water

1 cup sweetened vanilla almond milk or other nondairy alternative

½ teaspoon cinnamon

½ teaspoon salt

1 cup fresh berries

PREPARATION:

1. Using a fine strainer or sieve, rinse the quinoa well.

2. Add all the ingredients except the berries to a small pot and bring them to a low simmer.

3. Cover and continue to simmer for 15-20 minutes.

4. Serve quinoa warm or cold and top with fresh berries.

VARIATIONS:

▶ *Banana and Almond Butter Breakfast Quinoa (makes 2 servings):* In addition to the above, add ¼ teaspoon nutmeg and 1 teaspoon vanilla to the small pot of quinoa. Instead of berries, top each bowl with ½ tablespoon of chunky almond butter, ½ sliced banana, and ½ tablespoon pecans.

▶ *Leftover Vanilla Almond Quinoa Bowl (makes 2 servings):* Use any leftover cooked quinoa to make a breakfast bowl. Pour the vanilla almond milk and cinnamon (from the original recipe, above) into a pot and add ¼ teaspoon nutmeg and ¾ tablespoon maple syrup. Whisk over low heat until the ingredients are warm and thoroughly mixed. Top each serving with 1 tablespoon sliced almonds and ½ cup blueberries.

PER SERVING: 401 calories, 13 grams protein, 74 grams carbohydrates, 7 grams total fat

CHUNKY CINNAMON PEAR OATMEAL

PREP TIME: 5 min

COOK TIME: 5 min

TOTAL TIME: 10 min

MAKES 1 SERVING

Loaded with amazing health benefits from lowering blood sugar to treating muscle spasms, the common cold and erectile dysfunction, cinnamon is a powerhouse. We've paired it with pears (yes, on purpose) for a delicious breakfast that will set the tone for an awesome day.

INGREDIENTS:

½ cup gluten-free oats

1 cup sweetened vanilla almond milk or non-dairy beverage of choice

1 tablespoon almond butter

1 teaspoon milled flaxseed

½ small pear, peeled and diced

1 tablespoon sliced almonds, for topping

dash cinnamon

PREPARATION:

1. Combine the oats and almond milk in a small pot over medium-low heat.

2. Bring to a simmer, stirring frequently for a few minutes.

3. Once the oatmeal begins to thicken, add the almond butter, milled flaxseed, and diced pears, and stir for another few minutes.

4. Remove from heat and serve. Top with almonds and a dash of cinnamon, and enjoy!

VARIATIONS:

▶ *Maple Pecan Oatmeal (make 2 servings):* Add ½ cup more oats, 1 tablespoon pecan meal, and 1 cup water to the pot in step 1 above. Top each serving with ½ banana (sliced), ¼ cup blueberries, 1 tablespoon pecans, and 1 tablespoon maple syrup.

▶ *Quick Oatmeal Protein Bowl (makes 1 serving):* Mix a large banana, ¼ teaspoon cinnamon, 1 cup sweetened vanilla almond milk, 2 tablespoons chia seeds, and 1 scoop 22 Days Plant-Protein Powder (the flavor of your choice) in a blender until smooth. In a small pot, combine protein mix and ½ cup oats over medium-low heat for five minutes or until warm. Top with fresh berries and raw nuts.

PER SERVING: 499 calories, 12 grams protein, 74 grams carbohydrates, 18 grams total fat

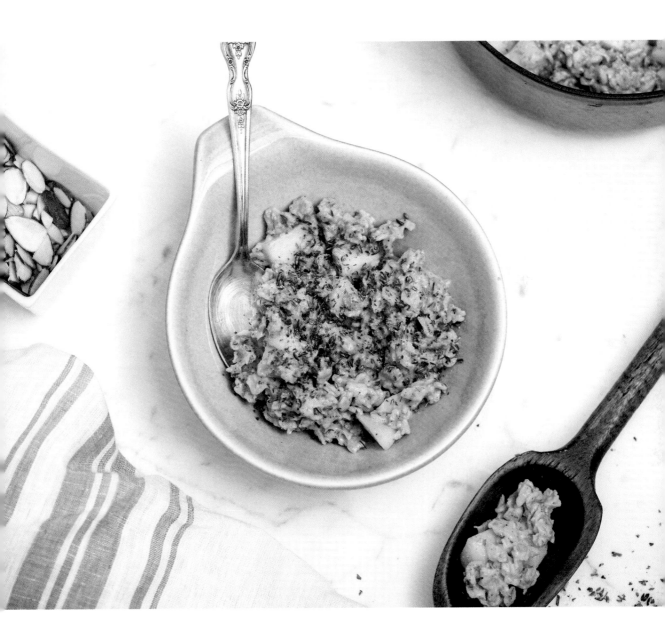

MUESLI

PREP TIME: 5 min

COOK TIME: 10 min

TOTAL TIME: 15 min (does not include overnight refrigeration)

MAKES 8 SERVINGS (¾ CUP EACH)

Full of nutrients and low in fat, muesli is incredibly versatile and delicious and a great way to start your day. We've added golden raisins and cranberries for a natural sweetness, and the fiber will fill you up without filling you out.

INGREDIENTS:

3⅔ cups rolled oats

½ cup dried cranberries

⅓ cup golden raisins

⅓ cup sunflower seeds

⅓ cup pumpkin seeds

⅓ cup sliced almonds

¼ cup walnuts, chopped

¼ cup cashews, chopped

½ teaspoon ground cinnamon

PREPARATION:

1. Preheat oven to 350F.

2. Place oats on baking sheet and bake for 5–10 minutes, until golden brown.

3. Remove the oats from the oven and let them cool completely.

4. In a large bowl, mix together the baked oats with the remaining ingredients. Store in an airtight container until ready to use.

5. To serve, pour about ¾ cup of muesli into a bowl with ½ cup of almond milk and enjoy! Feel free to top with fresh fruit of choice.

PER SERVING: 482 calories, 17 grams protein, 68 grams carbohydrates, 17 grams total fat

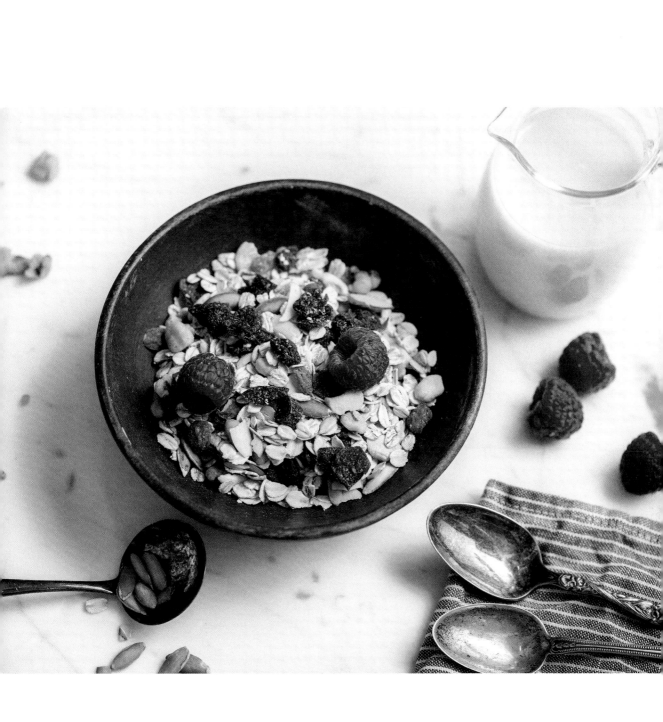

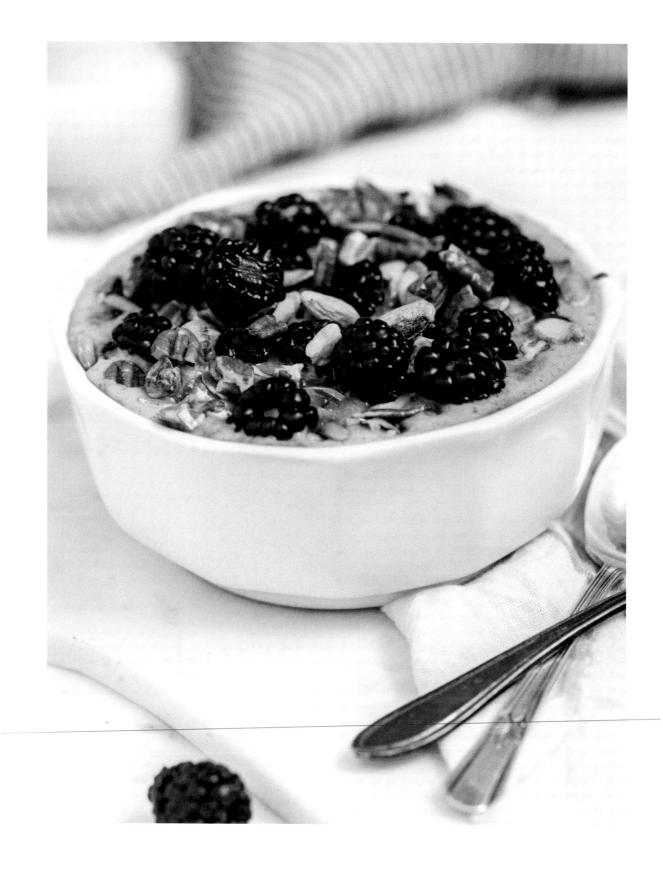

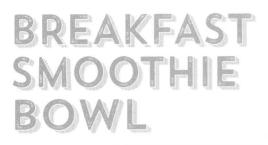

BREAKFAST SMOOTHIE BOWL

PREP TIME: 10 min

COOK TIME: 0 min

TOTAL TIME: 10 min

MAKES 1 SERVING

This bowl is loaded with nutrition and is very easy to make. Perfect for those mornings when you're on the run.

INGREDIENTS:

1 frozen banana

½ cup frozen blueberries

1 cup fresh spinach

¾ cup unsweetened almond milk

2 tablespoons pumpkin seeds

1 tablespoon pecans

1 tablespoon pistachios

6 fresh blackberries

PREPARATION:

1. Blend together banana, blueberries, spinach, and almond milk until mixture has reached smoothie consistency.

2. Pour smoothie into cereal bowl and sprinkle with pumpkin seeds, pecans, pistachios, and fresh blackberries.

PER SERVING: 429 calories, 11 grams protein, 62 grams carbohydrates, 19 grams total fat

CHOCOLATE DREAM SMOOTHIE

PREP TIME: 5 min

COOK TIME: 0 min

TOTAL TIME: 5 min

MAKES 1 SERVING

There's a reason chocolate is so popular. Unfortunately, most chocolate smoothies are loaded with sugar and devoid of nutrients. Here's a great recipe full of nutrition and taste without the added sugar.

INGREDIENTS:

1 cup sweetened vanilla almond milk

1 scoop 22 Days Chocolate Plant-Protein Powder

1 frozen banana or 1 banana and 1 cup ice

1 tablespoon almond butter

½ tablespoon cacao powder

¼ teaspoon vanilla extract

1 teaspoon vegan chocolate chips, for topping

PREPARATION:

1. Blend all the ingredients except chocolate chips until smooth.

2. Serve in a mason jar and top with chocolate chips.

PER SERVING: 450 calories, 22 grams protein, 57 grams carbohydrates, 16 grams total fat

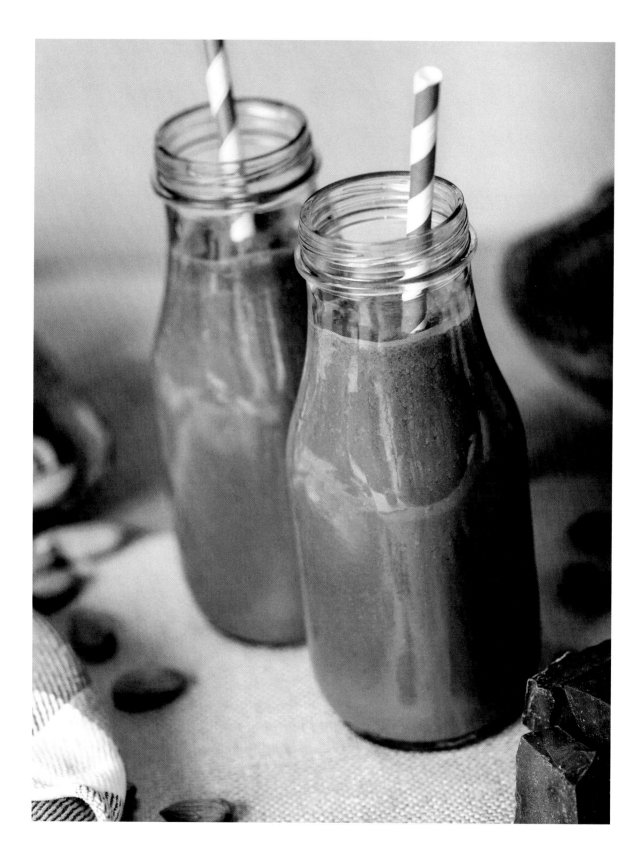

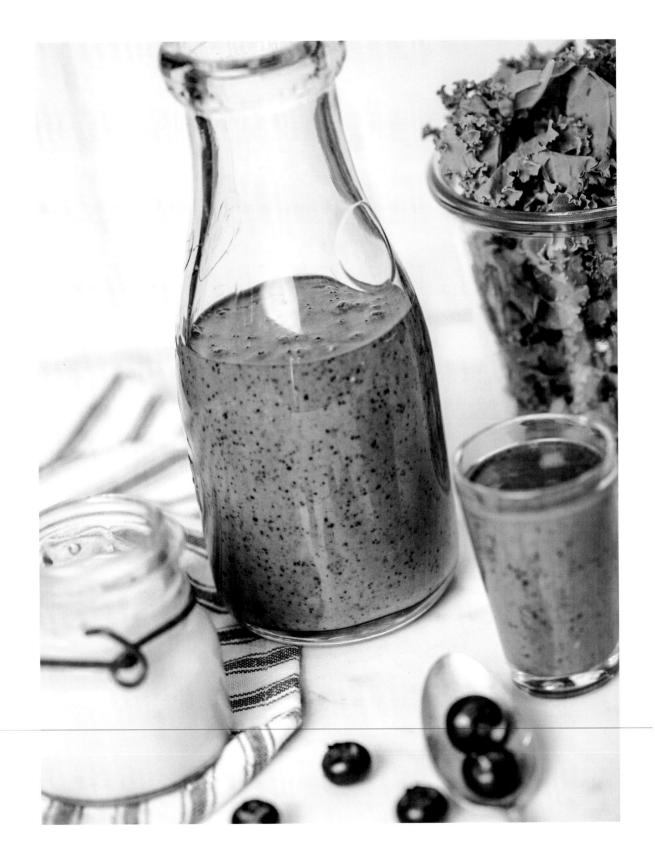

SWEET KALE SMOOTHIE

PREP TIME: 5 min
COOK TIME: 0 min
TOTAL TIME: 5 min

MAKES 1 SERVING

Kale and blueberries? you ask. Yes, this is an all-time favorite in our home, and we're sure it will be in yours too. I love this as a post-workout recovery shake, but it can also be used as a light meal and/or snack.

INGREDIENTS:

1 cup unsweetened almond milk

1 frozen banana

½ cup frozen blueberries

1 cup kale

1 heaping tablespoon sunflower butter

1 scoop 22 Days Plant-Protein Powder

PREPARATION:

1. Blend together all ingredients until smooth.

2. Pour into a glass and enjoy.

PER SERVING: 468 calories, 24 grams protein, 68 grams carbohydrates, 14 grams total fat

ENERGY BOOST

PREP TIME: 10 min

COOK TIME: 0 min

TOTAL TIME: 10 min

MAKES 1 SERVING

Beets are a great source of vitamin C, fiber and potassium and are known to increase nitric oxide in the body, which improves blood flow and helps with endurance and heart health.

INGREDIENTS:

1 green apple, cored

1 inch ginger, peeled

2 lemons, peeled

4 small beets

1 cup kale

2 large carrots

PREPARATION:

Juice all ingredients in a juicer, and enjoy!

PER SERVING: 406 calories, 12 grams protein, 97 grams carbohydrates, 2 grams total fat

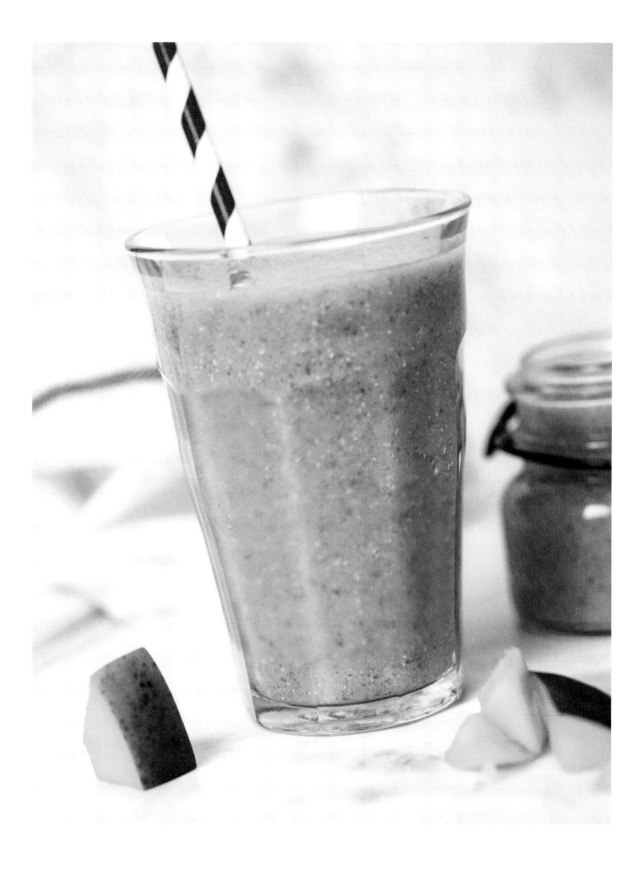

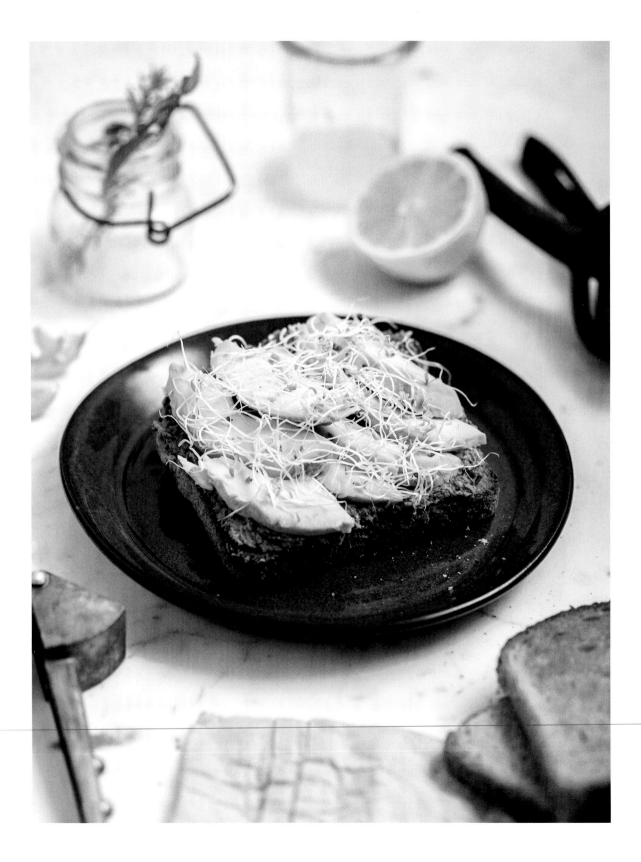

BLACK BEAN HUMMUS AVOCADO TARTINE

PREP TIME: 10 min

COOK TIME: 5 min

TOTAL TIME: 15 min

MAKES 2 SERVINGS

For the French, a tartine is an open-faced sandwich usually served with a spread. This one is a heart-healthy breakfast that is full of fiber, potassium, folate, and B_6. It will have you wondering how it could be so good and good for you at the same time.

INGREDIENTS:

1 15-ounce can black beans, drained and rinsed

1 clove garlic, minced

2 tablespoons tahini

1 lemon, juiced

1 teaspoon ground cumin

dash cayenne pepper (optional)

dash sea salt

dash ground black pepper

4 slices gluten-free vegan bread of choice

½ Hass avocado, halved, cored, peeled, and sliced

fresh sprouts, for garnish

PREPARATION:

1. In a food processor, combine the black beans, garlic, tahini, lemon juice, cumin, cayenne, salt, and pepper. Pulse until almost smooth.

2. Toast the bread and top it with the black bean spread, avocado, and sprouts.

3. Season with salt and pepper, to taste.

PER SERVING: 502 calories, 17 grams protein, 73 grams carbohydrates, 18 grams total fat

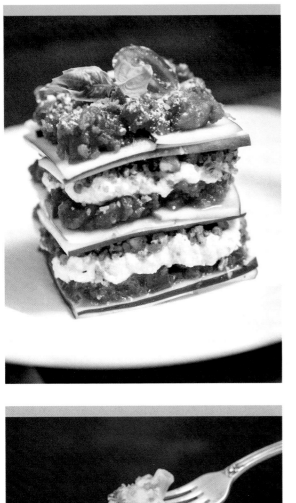

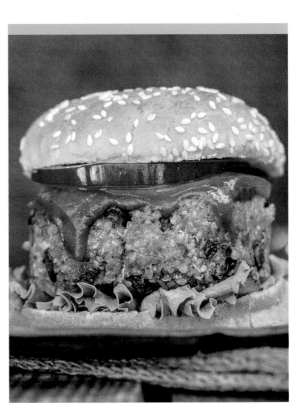

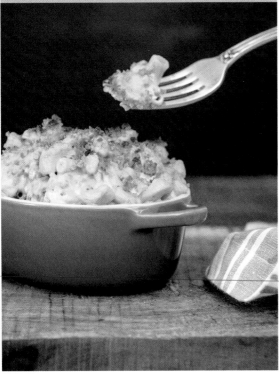

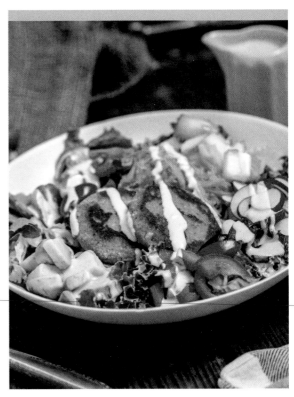

MAIN MEALS

MOST NIGHTS A WEEK, there's no time for dinner to be a decadent affair. But just because you're short on time doesn't mean your dinner needs to be short on flavor. And lunch is often crammed between the demands of a busy day. It's important to pause and refuel with nutrient-packed meals. All of our entrées are loaded with herbs and spices to wow your taste buds while your body gets plenty of vitamins and minerals. We've carefully organized these recipes so that whether you're in the mood for a lighter bite or a more indulgent comfort-food-style dinner, you'll be getting all of your nutrition while you lose weight, feel great, and get to know how delicious plant-based entrées can be.

Our Light Level 1 entrées, such as Avocado & Basil Cream Zucchini Noodles and Sweet Potato & Chickpea Soup, are lighter in calories and still rich in taste. Our Level 2 comfort foods, such as Mac 'n' Cheese and Cuban Brown Rice Bowl, will give you all the satisfaction of your favorites, and the extra satisfaction that comes along with meeting your weight goals. And our dips and sides, such as Mashed Cauliflower and Guacamole, round out your meals, giving you extra energy when you need it while maximizing flavor.

So have your friends over! Have your kids' friends over! Show the whole neighborhood just how delicious, how satisfying, how easy, how incredible plant-based eating can be!

LIGHT MEALS
(UNDER 300 CALORIES)

These meals are light and simple to leave you feeling satisfied but not stuffed. They're simple, easy-to-make, and easy-on-your-body dishes that are designed for a light yet deliciously nutritious meal.

When it comes to keeping lunch or dinner light, soup and a salad can be excellent selections. As an appetizer or a meal unto itself, you can enjoy a big bowl of veggies as a soup or salad. Warming and satisfying on a cold winter night—cool and refreshing on a hot summer day—soups and salads work for every season. Both can be served up hearty and full of grains and beans or lighter and full of carrots and greens. And the best part about making soups is that it's so easy to make twice as much and freeze individual portions for later.

Greens, greens, and more greens! There is no better way to achieve optimum intake of fresh veggies than through salads. Preparing salads can be quite easy, and with a little creativity, a few ingredients can go a very long way. And we love our salads when they are made with the tangiest dressings, like Creamy Cashew Balsamic Vinaigrette Dressing and Tahini Dressing.

In my house, we sometimes eat our soups blended smooth and creamy, like Sweet Potato & Chickpea Soup, or we might go for something a little more rustic, like Kale-Yeah Soup, full of satisfying bites. My grandmother used to make soup for us all the time, and I always loved it when she did. As I grew older, soup remained a perennial favorite, and I began to experiment with new recipes and flavors along with my wife, a fellow soup lover.

Whether you have a warm and tasty bowl of soup or a plate of bright, vibrant, freshly chopped veggies—either way, you'll be getting all your nutrients, and some delicious flavors too.

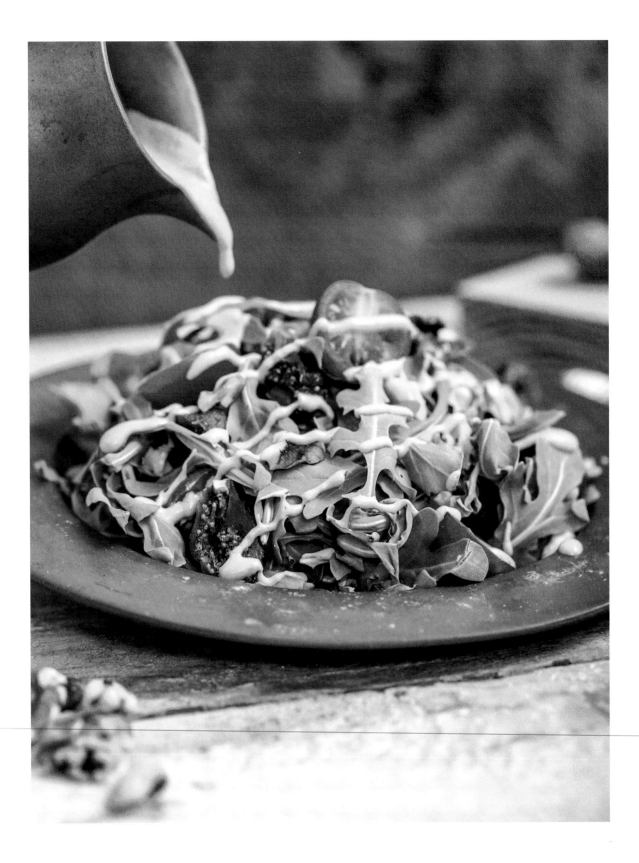

ARUGULA & FIG SALAD

PREP TIME: 10 min

COOK TIME: 0 min

TOTAL TIME: 10 min

MAKES 2 SERVINGS

Here's a quick and easy salad that doesn't lack in taste. Figs are a great source of fiber and can also help lower blood pressure, reduce the risk of macular degeneration and protect against breast cancer.

INGREDIENTS:

1 5-ounce package organic baby arugula

6 figs, washed and quartered

cherry tomatoes, washed and halved

¼ cup walnuts, roughly chopped

Creamy Cashew Balsamic Vinaigrette Dressing (see recipe on page 327)

(see recipe on page 327)

PREPARATION:

1. In a colander, thoroughly wash and drain the arugula.

2. In a serving dish, place the arugula and top with figs, tomatoes and walnuts.

3. Drizzle with dressing and serve!

PER SERVING WITH 2 TABLESPOONS OF DRESSING: 267 calories, 7 grams protein, 38 grams carbohydrates, 13 grams total fat

ASIAN SALAD WITH PEANUT SESAME DRESSING

PREP TIME: 20 min

COOK TIME: 0 min

TOTAL TIME: 20 min

MAKES 4 SERVINGS

Cabbage is full of vitamin K, may reduce the risk of cancer, and is loaded with vitamins and minerals. This Asian salad is incredibly savory while still being light. It's a crowd-pleaser and can be made in large portions for parties.

INGREDIENTS FOR PEANUT SESAME DRESSING:

2 tablespoons creamy peanut butter

2 tablespoons coconut aminos

2 tablespoons rice vinegar

1 tablespoon apple cider vinegar

1 tablespoon avocado oil or water

1 teaspoon maple syrup

2 teaspoons black sesame seeds

⅛ teaspoon ground garlic powder

⅛ teaspoon chili powder

INGREDIENTS FOR SALAD:

4 cups green or savoy cabbage, shredded

3 cups red cabbage, shredded

1 cup carrots, shredded

1 large red pepper, cored, seeded, and sliced

⅓ cup cashews, whole pieces and crushed, for garnish

black sesame seeds, for garnish

PREPARATION:

1. Prepare dressing by whisking together all dressing ingredients. To thin dressing, add 1 tablespoon of water at a time until desired consistency is reached. Taste and adjust seasoning as needed. Dressing can be made in advance and stored in an airtight glass container in the refrigerator for up to 1 week.

2. In a mixing bowl, place the cabbages, carrots, and peppers. Add the dressing and toss together to combine.

3. Transfer salad to a serving bowl, garnish with cashews and sesame seeds, and enjoy!

PER SERVING: 237 calories, 7 grams protein, 26 grams carbohydrates, 15 grams total fat

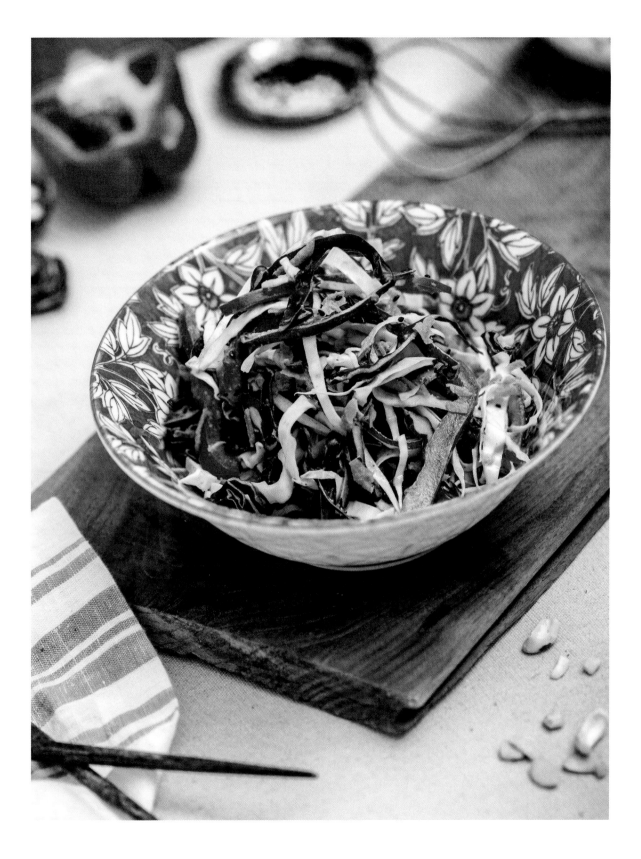

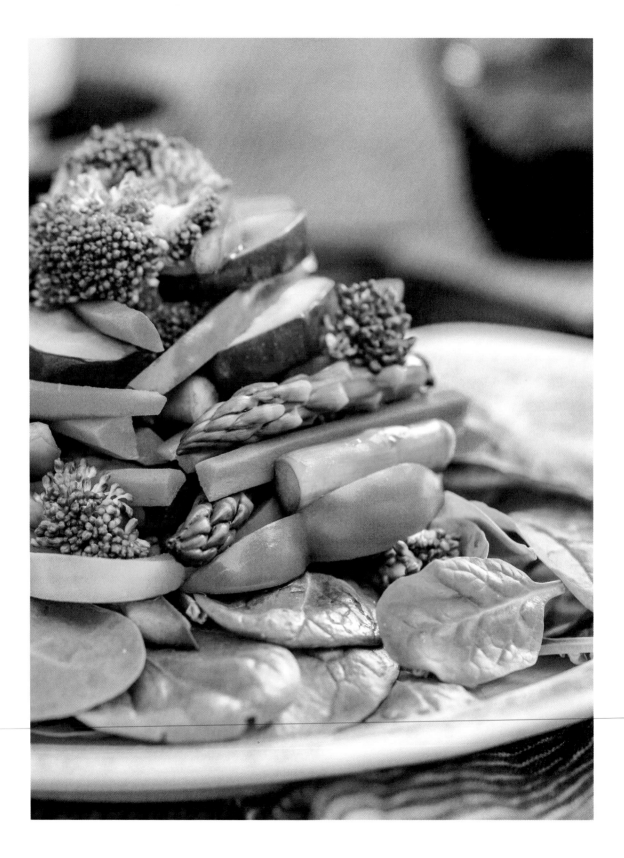

BALSAMIC VEGETABLES

PREP TIME: 15 min

COOK TIME: 10 min

TOTAL TIME: 25 min

MAKES 4 SERVINGS

Looking for an easy way to add more veggies to your diet? Look no further. This dish is extremely versatile and a family favorite anytime of the year. Feel free to add in seasonal veggies to keep things fresh and exciting.

INGREDIENTS:

1 bunch asparagus, cut into 2-inch pieces

1 head of broccoli, chopped into small florets

4 zucchini, sliced, then chopped in half

1 green pepper, sliced

1 orange or red pepper, sliced

4 large carrots, chopped and sliced into spears

6 tablespoons balsamic vinegar

4 tablespoons coconut aminos

sea salt, to taste

ground black pepper, to taste

bunch of spinach

PREPARATION:

1. Steam all veggies except the spinach for 7–10 minutes.

2. Drain the veggies and toss in a mixing bowl with vinegar and coconut aminos. Sprinkle with salt and pepper.

3. Serve the dressed veggies over a bed of spinach, and enjoy.

PER SERVING: 128 calories, 6 grams protein, 25 grams carbohydrates, 1 gram total fat

BEET SALAD WITH PEAR AND CANDIED PECANS

PREP TIME: 15 min

COOK TIME: 30 min

TOTAL TIME: 45 min

MAKES 4 SERVINGS

Beets and cheese! Arugula is loaded with vitamins A and K and includes vitamin C, folate, and fiber, all of which have very few calories and make for a perfect combination of flavor and nutrition.

INGREDIENTS:

4 small beets

1 5-ounce package organic baby arugula or spinach

1 ripe pear, sliced thin lengthwise

¼ cup Cashew Cheese
(see recipe on page 320)

½ cup Candied Pecans
(see recipe on page 237)

microgreens, for garnish

Balsamic Vinaigrette Dressing (see recipe on page 311)

PREPARATION:

1. Scrub the beets clean and place them in a steamer basket, then steam for about 30 minutes, until fork tender.

2. Let the beets cool, then gently rub off the skin. Cut into slices and set aside.

3. On a serving plate, arrange the arugula or spinach. Top with the sliced beets, pear, 2 teaspoon-size scoops of Cashew Cheese, Candied Pecans, and microgreens.

4. Drizzle with dressing, and serve!

PER SERVING WITH 2 TABLESPOONS OF DRESSING: 143 calories, 4 grams protein, 20 grams carbohydrates, 6 grams total fat

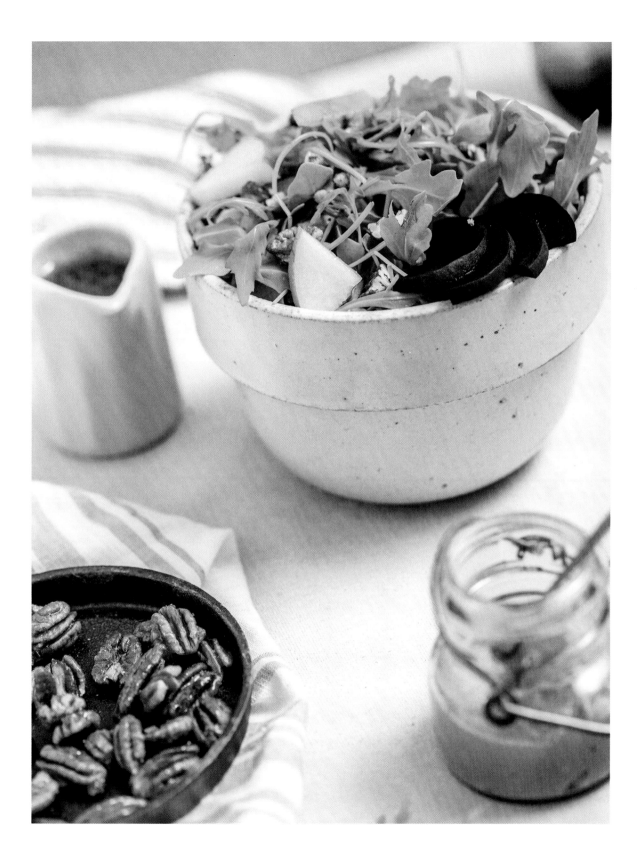

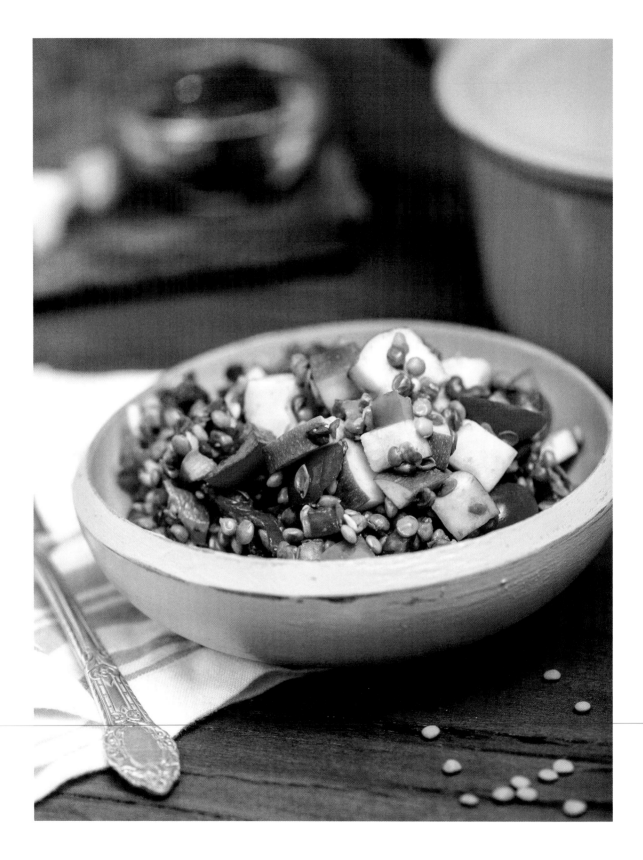

BELUGA LENTIL SALAD

PREP TIME: 10 min

COOK TIME: 25 min

TOTAL TIME: 35 min

MAKES 2 SERVINGS

Black lentils (like beluga) are delicate in flavor and a little more firm than regular lentils. These tiny beauties are loaded with protein and an impressive amount of vitamins and minerals, which make for a perfect meal anytime of the day.

INGREDIENTS:

1 cup beluga lentils, rinsed

4 tablespoons balsamic vinegar

2 tablespoons lime juice

1 zucchini, chopped

¼ cup sun-dried tomatoes, chopped

¼ cup grape tomatoes, sliced

¼ cup chopped red and green pepper

sea salt, to taste

ground black pepper, to taste

1 garlic clove, minced (optional)

PREPARATION:

1. Boil the lentils in 4 cups of water, then reduce the heat to simmer until the lentils are tender to the bite, about 20–25 minutes.

2. In a large mixing bowl, toss together all other ingredients. Then gently fold in the lentils.

3. Allow the salad to cool before serving. (Salad is best when refrigerated.)

PER SERVING: 204 calories, 14 grams protein, 36 grams carbohydrates, 1 gram total fat

BRUSSELS SPROUTS SALAD

PREP TIME: 20 min

COOK TIME: 0 min

TOTAL TIME: 20 min

MAKES 4 SERVINGS

This is one of my personal favorite salads. Brussels sprouts are an excellent source of vitamins C, B_6, and K, folate, manganese, fiber, potassium, and iron, just to name a few. This salad is easy to make and loaded with health benefits.

INGREDIENTS:

1 pound brussels sprouts (about 25–30), washed, stems trimmed (approximately 4 cups shredded)

Balsamic Vinaigrette Dressing (see recipe on page 311)

1 Hass avocado, halved, cored, peeled, and chopped

⅓ cup chopped walnuts

⅓ cup cranberries

Creamy Cashew Balsamic Vinaigrette Dressing (see recipe on page 327)

PREPARATION:

1. Use a sharp knife to slice the brussels sprouts in half, lengthwise. Place the halves cut side down on a cutting board. Then cut each half several times vertically from the top to the base. Can also use a mandolin slicer.

2. Transfer the shredded brussels sprouts to a mixing bowl and toss together with about ¼ cup of Balsamic Vinaigrette Dressing or desired amount until well combined.

3. On a serving platter or 4 individual plates, place a layer of shredded brussels sprouts and top with avocado, walnuts, and cranberries.

4. Drizzle Creamy Cashew Balsamic Vinaigrette Dressing and serve!

PER SERVING WITH 2 TABLESPOONS OF CREAMY CASHEW BALSAMIC VINAIGRETTE DRESSING:
250 calories, 7 grams protein, 30 grams carbohydrates,
13 grams total fat

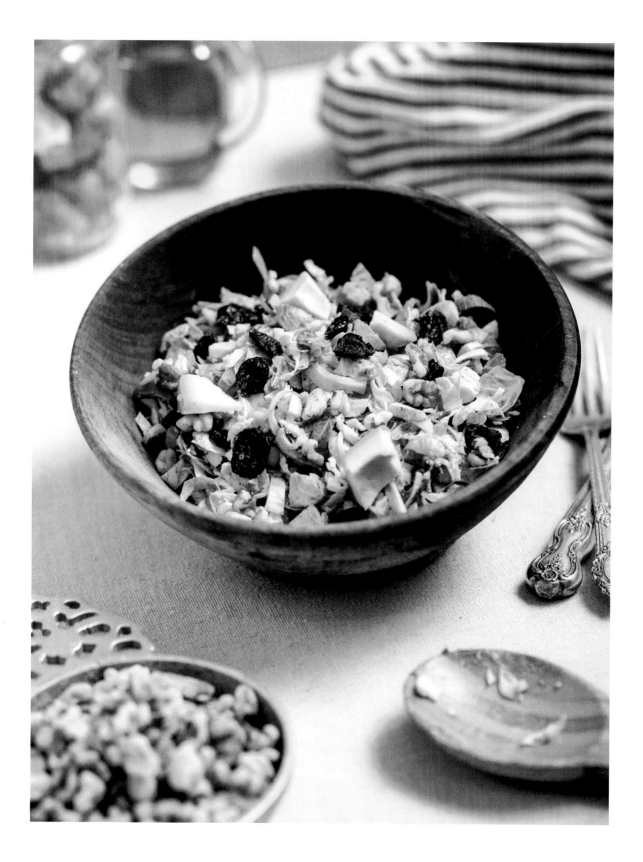

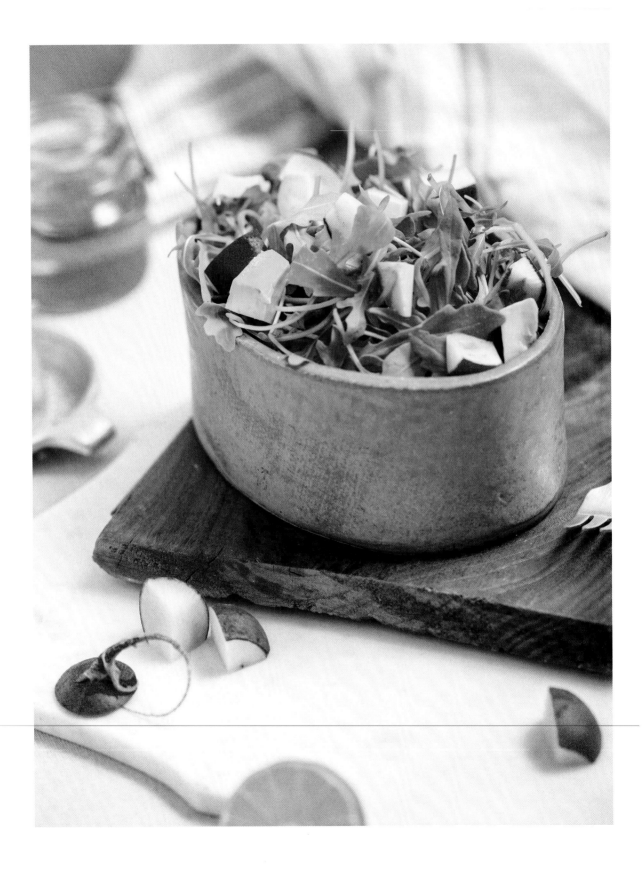

RADISH & AVOCADO SALAD

PREP TIME: 15 min

COOK TIME: 0 min

TOTAL TIME: 15 min

MAKES 2 SERVINGS

This salad is tiny but packs quite a bite. It's beautiful and delicious, but most of all, it's loaded with health benefits. Radishes help protect against cancers and viral infections while aiding in digestion. They're also known for eliminating toxins. Avocados are a great source of potassium, vitamins B_5, B_6, E, C, and K, and folate.

INGREDIENTS:

2 cups microgreens or arugula

2 cups radishes, diced

1 Hass avocado, halved, cored, peeled, and diced

1 tablespoon extra-virgin olive oil

1 lime, juiced

ground black pepper, to taste

sea salt, to taste

PREPARATION:

In a mixing bowl, gently toss together all the ingredients, and serve!

PER SERVING: 201 calories, 3 grams protein, 12 grams carbohydrates, 17 grams total fat

VEGGIE CHOPPED SALAD

PREP TIME: 30 min

COOK TIME: 0 min

TOTAL TIME: 30 min

MAKES 2 SERVINGS

This is an easy and delicious way to satisfy some of our recommended daily intake of veggies. It's quite simple to make, and for countless versions, we encourage creativity with ingredient selection by adding more veggies or swapping out some for others.

INGREDIENTS:

1 15-ounce can chickpeas, drained and rinsed

1 green bell pepper, washed, seeded, and finely chopped

1 red bell pepper, washed, seeded, and finely chopped

1 celery stalk, finely chopped

1 cup curly parsley, finely chopped

1 scallion, thinly sliced

2 handfuls spinach, chopped

parsley flakes, for garnish

Tahini Dressing (see recipe on page 344)

PREPARATION:

1. Drain and rinse the chickpeas.

2. In a mixing bowl, combine the chickpeas, peppers, celery, parsley, and scallions and toss to combine.

3. On a serving plate, place a layer of spinach, then top with chopped veggie mixture and garnish with parsley.

4. Drizzle salad with Tahini Dressing, and enjoy!

PER SERVING WITH 2 TABLESPOONS OF DRESSING: 252 calories, 12 grams protein, 38 grams carbohydrates, 7 grams total fat

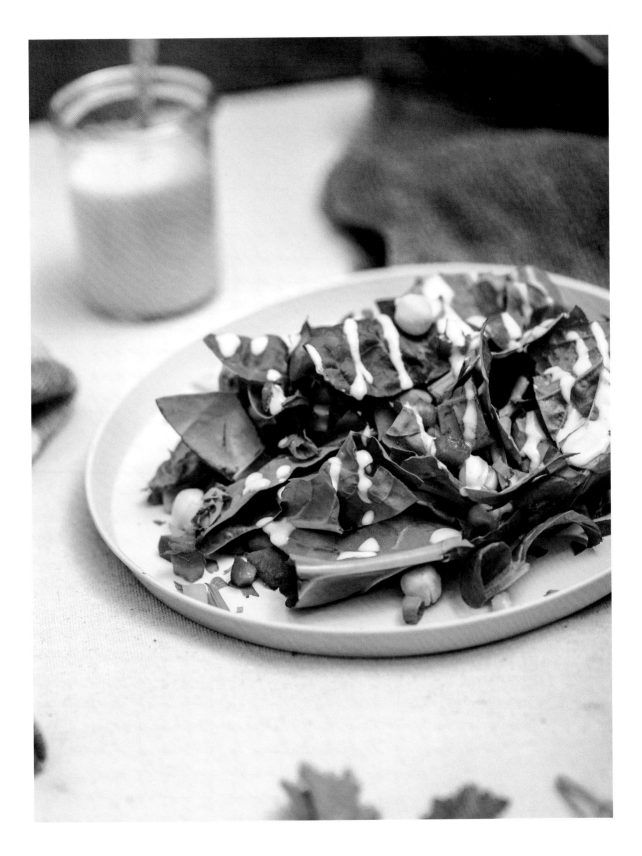

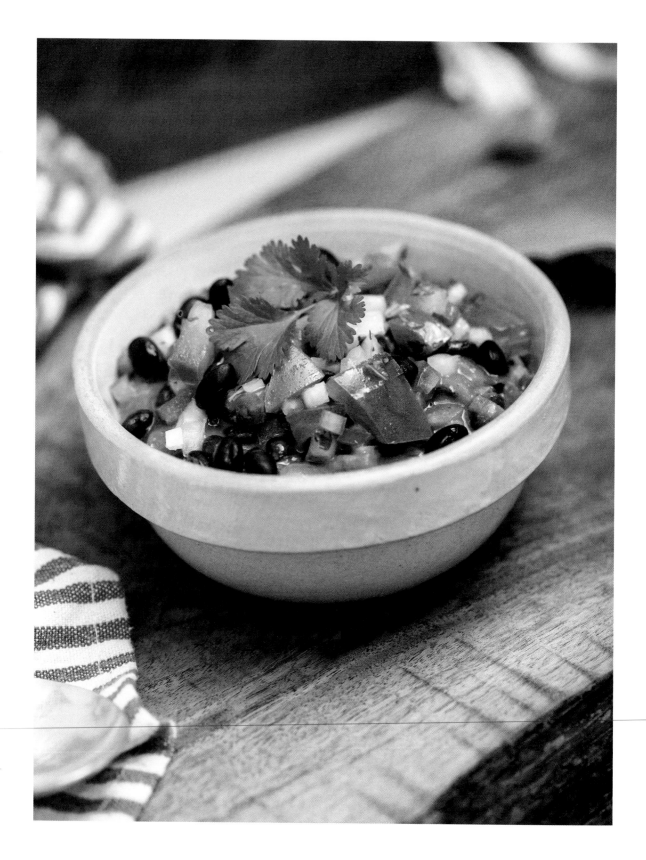

BLACK BEAN SOUP

PREP TIME: 10 min

COOK TIME: 2 hrs 30 min

TOTAL TIME: 2 hrs 40 min

MAKES 4 SERVINGS (ABOUT ¾ CUP)

This is a delicious and filling soup. Enjoy it with Pico de Gallo or with a side of brown rice and sliced avocado. Plan ahead and double this recipe, since it does take a long time to cook—and always tastes better the next day. Store leftovers in the refrigerator for up to a week or in the freezer for up to 3 months. When ready to enjoy again, reheat soup at a low simmer.

INGREDIENTS:

1 cup black beans, rinsed and presoaked overnight in 3 to 4 cups of water

1 tablespoon canola oil or oil of choice

1 small white onion, finely chopped (about ½ cup)

1 garlic clove, finely minced

¾ teaspoon sea salt or to taste

1 medium bell pepper, cored, seeded, and minced (about 1 cup)

1 tablespoon ground cumin

Pico de Gallo (see recipe on page 249)

PREPARATION:

1. Rinse and drain the beans.

2. In a large pot, add beans and enough water to barely cover them. Bring to a boil.

3. Reduce to medium-low heat, cover the pot and let simmer for up to 2 hours, stirring occasionally and skimming off any white foam that rises to the top. Add water if the beans seem too dry.

4. When the beans are just about tender, heat oil in a skillet over medium-high and sauté onion and garlic with a pinch of salt for 5 minutes or until onion is translucent. Stir in the peppers, cumin, and more sea salt and continue to cook.

5. Once the vegetables have softened, stir them into the pot of beans and taste to adjust seasoning, if necessary.

6. Continue to cook for another 30 minutes. The goal is to reach a creamy consistency, so let the beans cook until the soup base is thick, not watery.

7. When the beans are tender, serve and garnish with Pico de Gallo.

PER SERVING: 115 calories, 5 grams protein, 17 grams carbohydrates, 4 grams total fat

CHICKPEA SOUP

PREP TIME: 10 min

COOK TIME: 25 min

TOTAL TIME: 35 min

MAKES 6 SERVINGS

This is a quick and easy soup that takes just 35 minutes to prepare.

INGREDIENTS:

3 cups vegetable broth, unsalted or low sodium

3 cups water

2 medium Yukon or russet potatoes, peeled and cubed (about 4 cups)

1 small onion, peeled and halved

1 garlic clove, minced

1 tablespoon ground cumin

1½ teaspoons sea salt or to taste

½ teaspoon ground black pepper

2 15-ounce cans chickpeas, drained and rinsed (about 3–3½ cups)

PREPARATION:

1. To a large pot, add the 3 cups of vegetable broth and 3 cups of water and bring to a boil.

2. Add peeled and cubed potatoes and onion to boiling liquid.

3. Stir in the garlic, cumin, salt, and pepper.

4. Reduce to a simmer and cook uncovered for about 15 minutes, until potatoes are soft.

5. Transfer the onion and half of the potatoes with some broth to a blender. Add 1 can of chickpeas, and blend until smooth and creamy.

6. Transfer the soup mixture back into the pot and add the remaining chickpeas.

7. Continue to cook, stirring occasionally, at low heat for another 5–10 minutes. Taste and adjust the seasonings, if necessary.

8. Ladle the soup into bowls and enjoy! Feel free to add spinach or a green of your choice upon serving.

TIP: Leftovers can be stored in the refrigerator in an airtight container for a couple of days or in the freezer for up to 1 month.

PER SERVING: 191 calories, 7 grams protein, 36 grams carbohydrates, 2 grams total fat

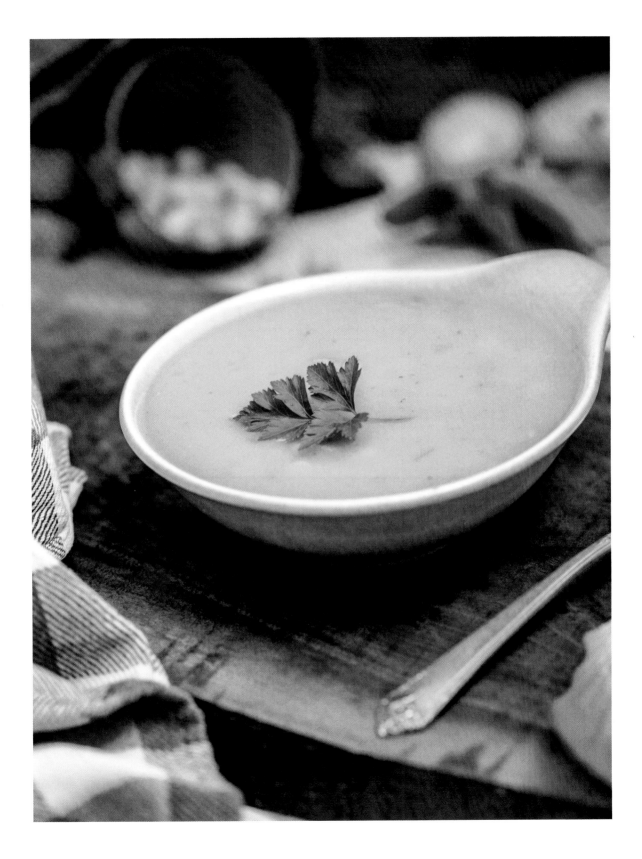

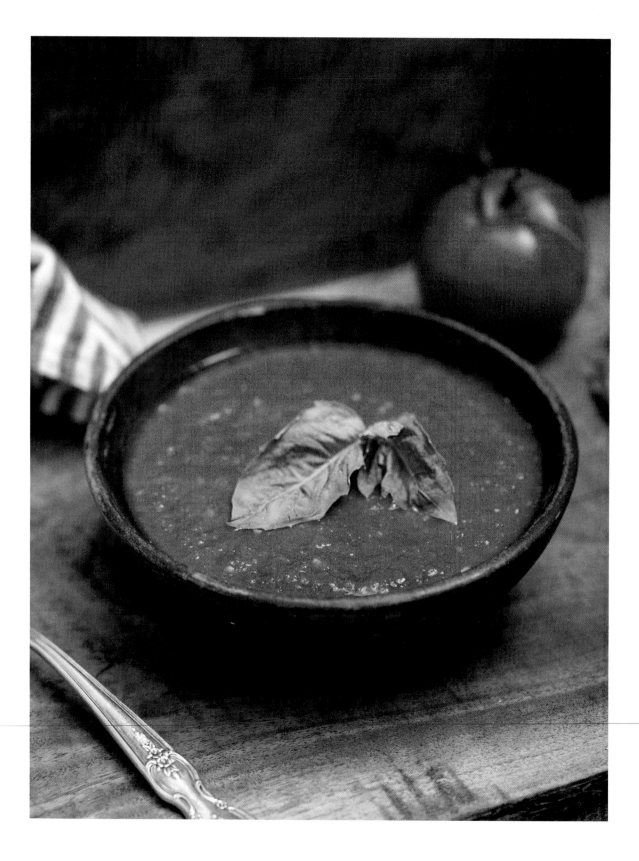

HEARTY TOMATO SOUP

PREP TIME: 10 min

COOK TIME: 30 min

TOTAL TIME: 40 min

MAKES 4 SERVINGS

This recipe can be enjoyed simply or garnished with sliced avocado and/or a scoop of Cashew Cheese.

INGREDIENTS:

8 large tomatoes, washed, cored, and roughly chopped

2 red peppers, washed, seeded, and chopped

¼ cup chopped basil leaves, set some aside for garnish

1 medium onion, chopped

1 garlic clove

½ teaspoon sea salt or to taste

dash cayenne pepper

basil, for garnish

(optional) Cashew Cheese (see recipe on page 320)

PREPARATION:

1. Add all soup ingredients to a blender and blend in batches until smooth.

2. Pour sauce in a large pot and cook at medium-low heat, stirring often, for 25–30 minutes, skimming off any foam that rises to the top. Sauce will darken as it cooks. Taste and adjust seasoning, if necessary.

3. To serve, top with a heaping tablespoon of Cashew Cheese (optional) and garnish with fresh basil—and enjoy!

TIP: Store leftovers in an airtight container in the fridge for up to 10 days or in the freezer for a few months. The soup is best when stored in single-portion-size containers to prolong freshness. This way you only touch the soup you're going to use.

PER SERVING: 75 calories, 3 grams protein, 16 grams carbohydrates, 1 gram total fat

KALE-YEAH SOUP

PREP TIME: 10 min

COOK TIME: 20 min

TOTAL TIME: 30 min

MAKES 6 SERVINGS

This kale soup is tasty and hearty, and it can easily become a go-to in your home. Kale is one of the most nutrient-rich foods around. It's loaded in vitamins A, B$_6$, C, K, manganese, calcium, potassium, magnesium, and the omega-3 linolenic acid.

INGREDIENTS:

1 tablespoon plus 1 teaspoon olive oil or oil of choice

1 small onion, chopped

1 garlic clove, minced

¾ teaspoon sea salt or to taste

1 small head cauliflower, trimmed and cut into florets

1 large bunch lacinato kale, destemmed and roughly chopped, reserve 1 to 2 cups for kale chip garnish

6 cups vegetable broth, unsalted or low sodium

PREPARATION:

1. Preheat oven to 350F and line a sheet pan with parchment paper.

2. In a large pot, heat 1 tablespoon of oil over medium-high heat, and sauté the onions with garlic and a pinch of sea salt until the onions become translucent.

3. Add the cauliflower and about ½ teaspoon sea salt and continue to cook for about 5 minutes.

4. Add the kale, except for 1–2 cups reserved for kale chips. Add the vegetable broth and bring to a boil.

5. Simmer for 10–15 minutes until the cauliflower becomes tender.

6. To make the kale chips, thoroughly dry the remaining kale, toss with 1 teaspoon of olive oil and the rest of the sea salt and bake for 20 minutes or until crisp.

7. Let the soup slightly cool, then puree in a blender in batches until smooth and creamy.

8. Return the smooth soup to the pot and continue to simmer it at low heat for another few minutes. Taste the soup and adjust the seasoning, if necessary.

9. Ladle the soup into bowls, garnish with kale chips, and serve!

TIP: This soup is also delicious topped with Cheezy Kale Chips (see recipe on page 269).

PER SERVING: 71 calories, 4 grams protein, 12 grams carbohydrates, 2 grams total fat

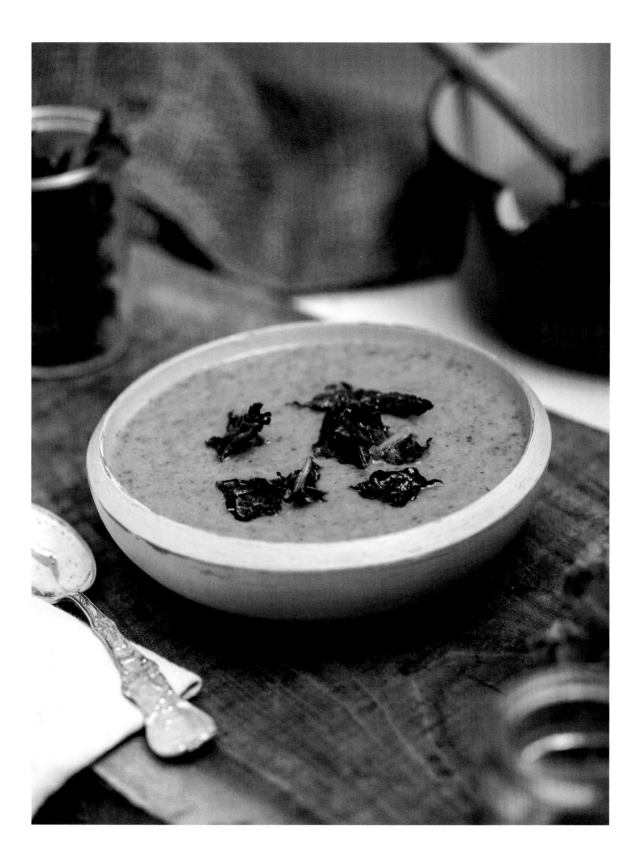

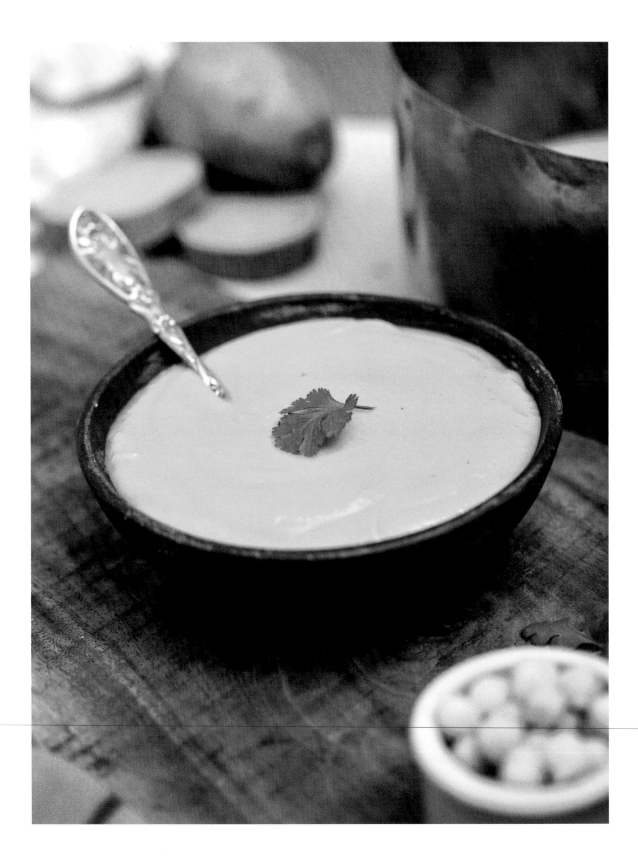

SWEET POTATO & CHICKPEA SOUP

PREP TIME: 5 min
COOK TIME: 30 min
TOTAL TIME: 35 min

MAKES 6 SERVINGS

This soup offers the perfect balance between sweet and savory, and it has a creamy consistency without added cream. Sweet potatoes, which rank low on the glycemic index scale, boast many beneficial nutrients. They are packed with calcium and vitamins A and C.

We enjoy this recipe as is and on occasion top it with our Crunchy Chickpeas (see recipe on page 242) or diced avocados for an added burst of flavor and creaminess.

INGREDIENTS:

1 tablespoon canola oil or oil of choice

1 small onion, diced

1 garlic clove, minced

½ teaspoon sea salt or to taste

2 medium sweet potatoes, cubed (about 4 cups)

2 teaspoons ground cumin

½ teaspoon ground black pepper

¼ teaspoon ground ginger

6 cups vegetable broth, unsalted or low sodium

1 15-ounce can chickpeas, rinsed and drained

microgreens, for garnish

PREPARATION:

1. In a large pot, heat the oil over medium-high heat and sauté the onions with garlic and a pinch of sea salt until the onions become translucent.

2. Add the sweet potatoes, sea salt, and spices and continue to cook for about 5 minutes.

3. Then add the vegetable broth and bring to a boil.

4. Simmer for 20–25 minutes until the sweet potatoes become tender. Remove the pot from the heat and allow the sweet potato–and-broth mixture to slightly cool.

5. Puree the mixture in a blender with chickpeas in batches until the soup is smooth and creamy.

6. Return the mixture to the pot and simmer over low heat for another few minutes. Taste the soup and add more seasonings, if necessary. To thin the soup, add more vegetable broth.

Recipe continues

7. Serve, garnished with micogreens, and enjoy!

TIP: Leftovers can be stored in the refrigerator for a couple of days or in the freezer for up to 1 month.

PER SERVING: 133 calories, 4 grams protein, 22 grams carbohydrates, 3 grams total fat

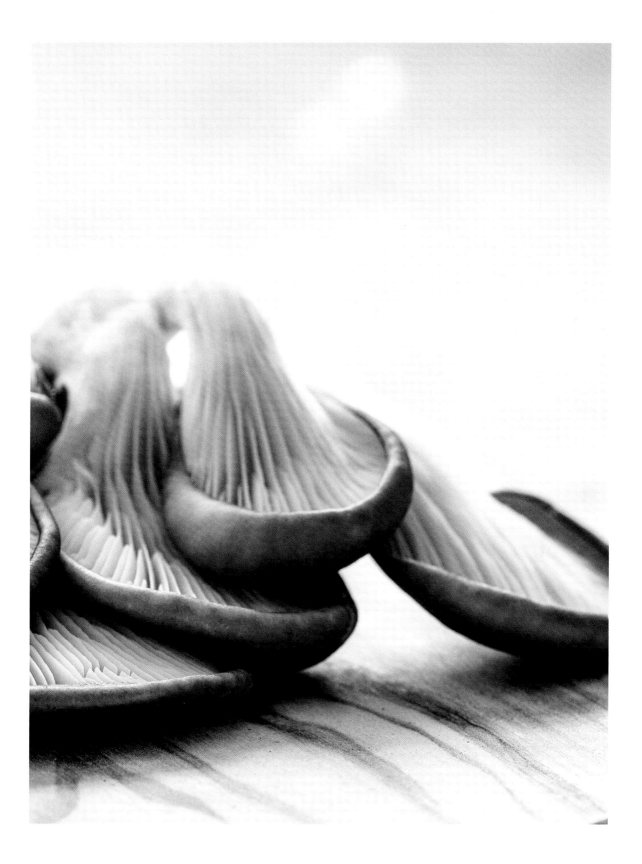

AVOCADO & BASIL CREAM ZUCCHINI NOODLES

PREP TIME: 15 min (does not include the Parmesan Cheese recipe)

COOK TIME: 10 min

TOTAL TIME: 25 min

MAKES 4 SERVINGS

This raw zucchini pasta is an incredible source of manganese, vitamin C, and fiber! It's a nutritiously powerful option to keep handy when you're short on time but don't want to sacrifice flavor.

INGREDIENTS:

2 large zucchini

1 Hass avocado, halved, pitted, and peeled

1 lemon, juiced

½ cup basil leaves, roughly chopped, set some aside for garnish

pinch of onion powder

pinch of garlic powder

¼–½ teaspoon sea salt or to taste

cherry tomatoes, halved, for garnish

Parmesan Cheese, to taste (see recipe on page 340)

PREPARATION:

1. Wash the zucchini, trim the ends, and carve the zucchini into curly strands, using a spiralizer or julienne peeler. Set aside while preparing sauce.

2. To prepare the sauce, process remaining ingredients, except the garnishes and Parmesan Cheese, in a food processor or blender until smooth.

3. Toss the zucchini noodles together with the sauce until fully coated.

4. Serve and garnish with cherry tomatoes, basil, and Parmesan Cheese and enjoy!

TIP: Avocados tend to oxidize quickly, so this recipe is best enjoyed immediately!

PER SERVING: 109 calories, 4 grams protein, 11 grams carbohydrates, 7 grams total fat

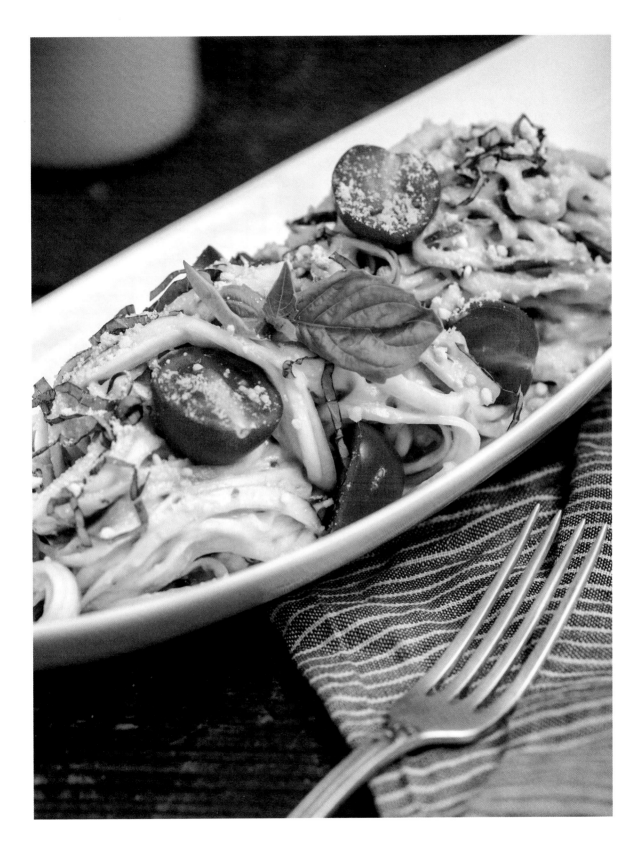

CHANA MASALA CHICKPEAS

PREP TIME: 10 min

COOK TIME: 20 min

TOTAL TIME: 30 min (does not include Go-To Tomato Sauce or Short-Grain Brown Rice prep time)

MAKES 4 SERVINGS

If planning your meals ahead of time, having the Grandma's Go-To Tomato Sauce and Short-Grain Brown Rice already prepared makes this dish quick and so much easier to make. Another time-saving tip is to have all the spices measured and combined in a small bowl, ready for when you decide to make this fragrant and warming Indian-inspired meal.

INGREDIENTS:

1 cup of Grandma's Go-To Tomato Sauce (see recipe on page 331)

2 cups cooked Short-Grain Brown Rice (see recipe on page 319)

1 teaspoon minced garlic

½ teaspoon sea salt, or to taste

1 tablespoon ground cumin

¼ teaspoon garam masala

1 teaspoon ground coriander

1 teaspoon smoked paprika

½ teaspoon paprika

¼ teaspoon ground turmeric

1 teaspoon ground ginger

⅛ teaspoon cayenne pepper (optional)

2 15-ounce cans chickpeas, drained and rinsed (about 3 cups)

1 lime, quartered, for garnish

fresh parsley flakes, or cilantro, for garnish

PREPARATION:

1. Prepare tomato sauce and brown rice. (Can be prepared ahead of time.)

2. If you have prepared the tomato sauce ahead of time, heat it in a large saucepan over medium heat.

3. Stir in the garlic, the salt, and all the spices and let the ingredients cook for a few minutes.

4. Raise the heat to medium-high. Add the chickpeas and stir until well combined.

5. Reduce to a simmer and cook for about 10–15 minutes, stirring often, to allow the flavors to blend together. Taste and adjust seasoning, if necessary.

6. Serve Chana Masala with brown rice, and garnish with a lime wedge and parsley flakes.

TIP: Leftovers can be stored in an airtight container in the refrigerator up to 4–5 days.

VARIATION:

► The Chana Masala can also be enjoyed with steamed vegetables, or atop a baked potato instead of brown rice.

PER SERVING: 182 calories, 9 grams protein, 31 grams carbohydrates, 3 grams total fat

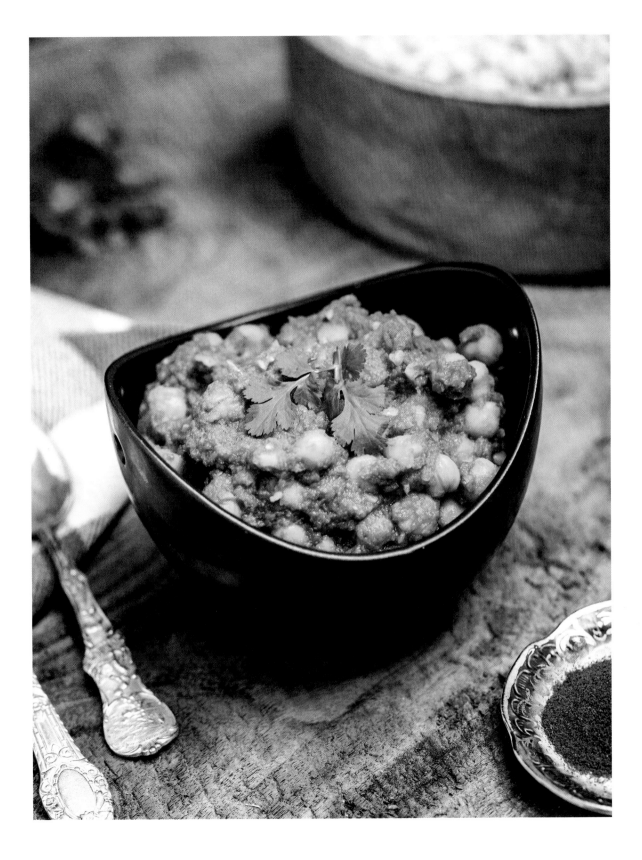

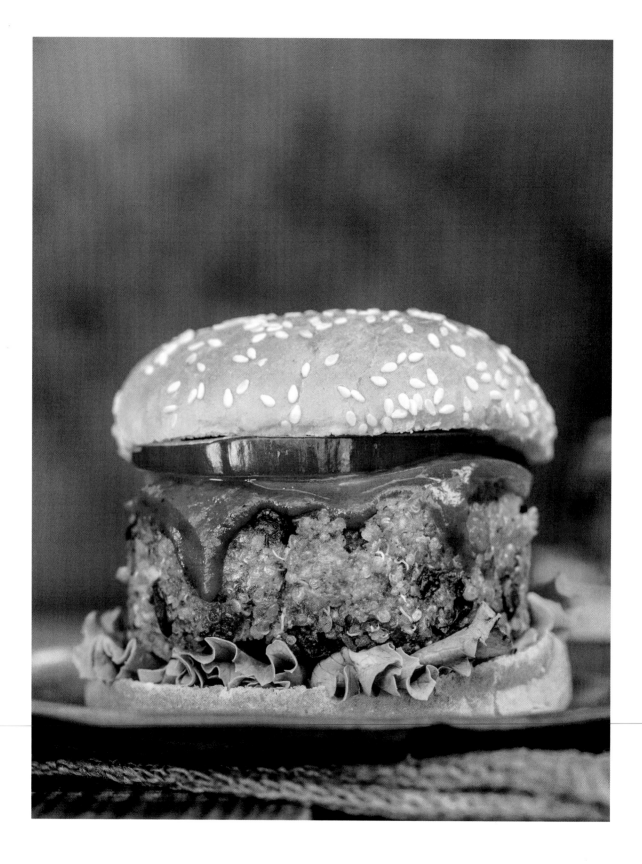

BLACK BEAN & QUINOA BURGER

PREP TIME: 15 min

COOK TIME: 55 min

TOTAL TIME: 70 min (does not include Black Beans cook time)

MAKES 4 PATTIES

You don't have to give up burgers in order to achieve optimal health! These burgers are as delicious as they are nutritious. So go ahead, plan the next party and treat your friends to the gift of health without sacrifice.

INGREDIENTS:

⅓ small onion, diced

1½ cup Black Beans, cooked (see recipe on page 315) or use canned, rinsed and drained

1½ cups cooked Quinoa (see recipe on page 343)

¼ cup minced fresh parsley

2 tablespoons flax meal

1 teaspoon ground cumin

1 teaspoon ground coriander

1 teaspoon lemon juice

4 tablespoons gluten-free bread crumbs

3 tablespoons quinoa flour

1 teaspoon baking powder

4 tablespoons water

½ teaspoon sea salt or to taste

oil of choice (if using a skillet)

PREPARATION:

1. Preheat oven to 400F and prepare a baking sheet lined with parchment paper.

2. In a food processor, process the onions and ½ of the Black Beans.

3. Scoop the mixture into a bowl and mix well with the remaining ingredients.

4. Create patties with the palms of your hands. Then place them on a baking sheet.

5. Bake for about 30 minutes, flipping halfway through.

TIP: If you're pressed for time, the patties can be cooked on a lightly greased skillet, with the oil of your choice, over medium heat for a few minutes on each side or until golden. Leftovers can be stored in an airtight container in the refrigerator for a few days or in the freezer for a few months.

PER SERVING: 232 calories, 11 grams protein, 39 grams carbohydrates, 4 grams total fat

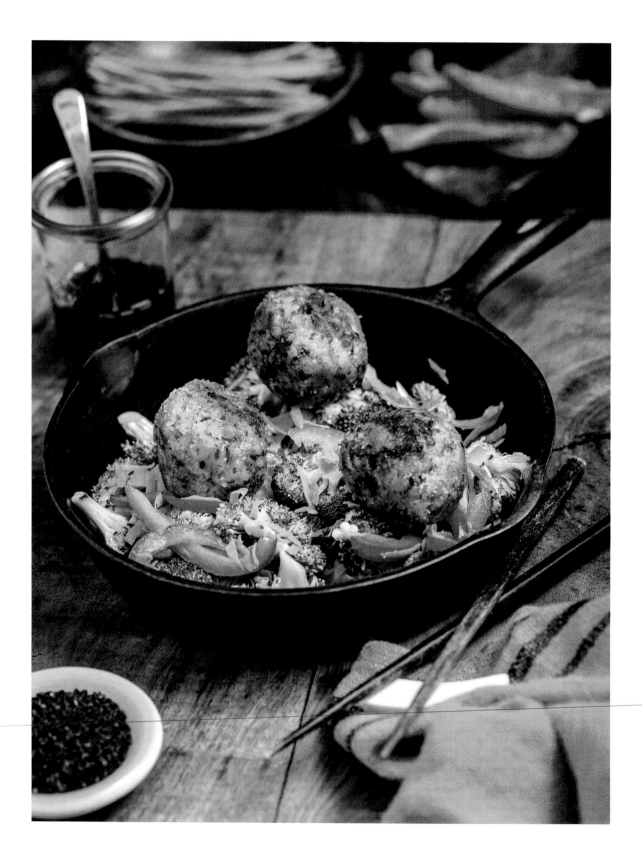

TERIYAKI VEGGIE BOWL WITH MEATLESS BALLS

PREP TIME: 25 min
COOK TIME: 75 min
TOTAL TIME: 100 min

MAKES 4 SERVINGS (20 MEATLESS MEATBALLS)

Teriyaki is one of those flavors we all crave sometimes. When we do, this bowl is the answer. It's quick and easy, and it can easily be modified to serve more. This is another great way to introduce new veggies to kids in a way they're sure to love.

INGREDIENTS FOR MEATLESS BALLS:

2 tablespoons canola oil, for skillet

2 cups mushrooms, washed, and chopped

1 small onion, diced (about ½ cup)

1 clove garlic, minced

1 teaspoon sea salt or to taste

½ teaspoon ground cumin

1½ cups unsalted cooked Short-Grain Brown Rice (see recipe on page 319) or Quinoa (see recipe on page 343)

3 tablespoons gluten-free flour (brown rice flour)

¼ cup plus 2 tablespoons gluten-free bread crumbs, with ¼ cup reserved for coating

½ teaspoon dried parsley

½ teaspoon dried basil

¼ teaspoon ground black pepper or to taste

⅛ teaspoon dried oregano

INGREDIENTS FOR TERIYAKI SAUCE:

¼ cup coconut aminos teriyaki sauce

2 tablespoons rice vinegar

2 tablespoons water

2 tablespoons sliced scallions

INGREDIENTS FOR VEGGIE BOWL:

1 large head broccoli, cut into florets

1 cup shredded carrots

1 large red bell pepper, washed, seeded, and thinly sliced into long strips

sesame seeds, for garnish

PREPARATION:

1. Prepare the Meatless Meatballs: Heat 1 tablespoon of oil in a large skillet over medium-high heat and sauté the mushrooms, onion, garlic, dash of salt, and cumin until soft. Set aside to cool.

2. In a food processor, add the mushroom mixture with the brown rice, flour, 2 tablespoons bread crumbs, parsley, basil, pepper and oregano and pulse until well combined.

Recipe continues

3. Coat with the remaining bread crumbs.

4. Using your hands, form about 20 tablespoon-sized meatballs.

5. Cook meatballs in a warm skillet, with the remaining 1 tablespoon of oil, over medium-high heat for about 5 minutes until golden brown. While cooking the meatballs, roll them in the pan to evenly brown them. Transfer the meatballs to a bowl and set aside.

6. Make the Teriyaki Sauce: Whisk all the sauce ingredients together and set the sauce aside until ready to use.

7. Prepare the Veggie Bowl: To the skillet, add the broccoli florets, carrots, red pepper strips, and ½ of the prepared teriyaki sauce. Cover the skillet and cook the veggies over medium heat for about 10 minutes, until tender. Add the Meatless Meatballs and the remaining Teriyaki Sauce and gently stir together. Cover and cook over medium-low heat for another few minutes.

8. Serve, top with sesame seeds, and enjoy!

TIP: Leftovers can be stored in the refrigerator for up to 2 days.

PER SERVING: 269 calories, 6 grams protein, 45 grams carbohydrates, 9 grams total fat

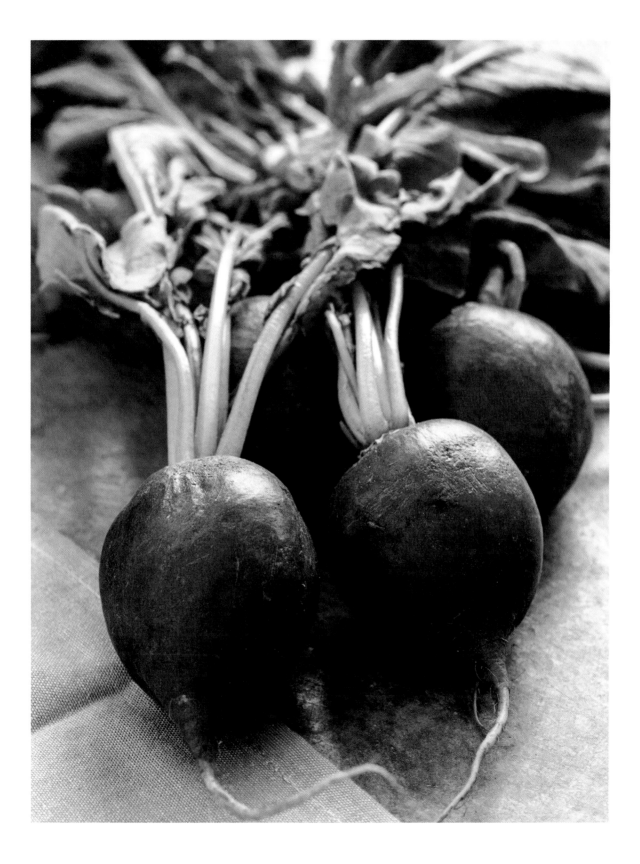

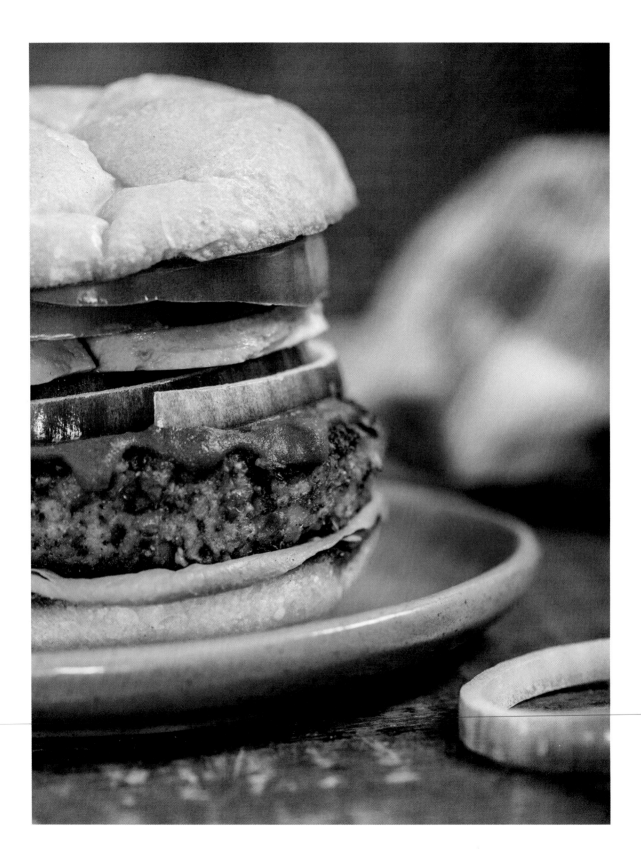

WALNUT BEAN BURGERS

PREP TIME: 20 min
COOK TIME: 60 min
TOTAL TIME: 80 min

MAKES 8 PATTIES

We love these Walnut Bean Burgers as part of a burger bar at home and offer them to our family with choices of toppings, sides, and different homemade breads for an exciting dining experience that nourishes from the inside out.

INGREDIENTS:

1 cup cooked Quinoa, cooked (see recipe on page 343)

1 cup Walnut Meat (see recipe on page 347)

1 15-ounce can pinto beans, rinsed and drained (about 1½ cups)

2 tablespoons onion, finely diced

1 clove garlic, minced

½ teaspoon sea salt or to taste

ground black pepper, to taste

PREPARATION:

1. Preheat oven to 400F and lightly grease a baking sheet or line it with parchment paper.

2. Place the cooked and slightly cooled Quinoa in a large mixing bowl.

3. Prepare the Walnut Meat and spoon it into the bowl.

4. In a food processor, pulse the pinto beans a few times, making sure not to overblend. Add the pinto beans to the Quinoa and Walnut Meat. Add the onions, garlic, salt, and pepper and mix all the ingredients together until well combined. Taste and adjust seasonings if necessary.

5. Divide the mixture into 8 portions and firmly shape each portion into a patty. Place the patties on the baking sheet.

6. Bake the patties for 20 minutes. Flip them carefully and bake for another 10–15 minutes.

7. Serve the burgers on your bread of choice with desired toppings. Some topping ideas: avocados, tomatoes, Cashew Cheese (see recipe on page 320), or BBQ Sauce (see recipe on page 312). Or serve the patties with a mixed green salad.

TIP: If pressed for time, cook the burgers in a skillet lightly greased with the oil of your choice over medium-high heat for about 4 minutes per side. The patties also can be prepped and stored in the refrigerator for up to 2 days or in the freezer, in freezer bags layered with parchment paper, for up to 2 months.

PER SERVING: 205 calories, 7 grams protein, 23 grams carbohydrates, 10 grams total fat

ROASTED BUTTERNUT SQUASH & QUINOA

PREP TIME: 15 min

COOK TIME: 25 min

TOTAL TIME: 40 min

MAKES 4 SERVINGS

This salad can be enjoyed warm or cold, and it is one of my lunchtime favorites because it's a complete protein source with just the right amount of flavor and crunch. We prepare this dish over the weekend, and have it ready to go in the fridge for weekday power lunches.

INGREDIENTS:

1 large butternut squash, peeled and diced

1 cup cooked Quinoa (see recipe on page 343)

1 Hass avocado, halved, pitted, and chopped into cubes

1 small lemon, juiced

sea salt, to taste

ground black pepper, to taste

¼ cup pumpkin seeds (pepitas)

PREPARATION:

1. Preheat oven to 350F. Steam the squash for 5–7 min. Scatter the squash bits over a parchment-lined baking sheet and roast in the oven for 10–15 minutes or until the edges are slightly browned.

2. In a mixing bowl, toss together the squash, quinoa, avocado, lemon juice, salt, and pepper. Transfer to a serving dish, sprinkle with pepitas and enjoy.

PER SERVING: 256 calories, 7 grams protein, 40 grams carbohydrates, 10 grams total fat

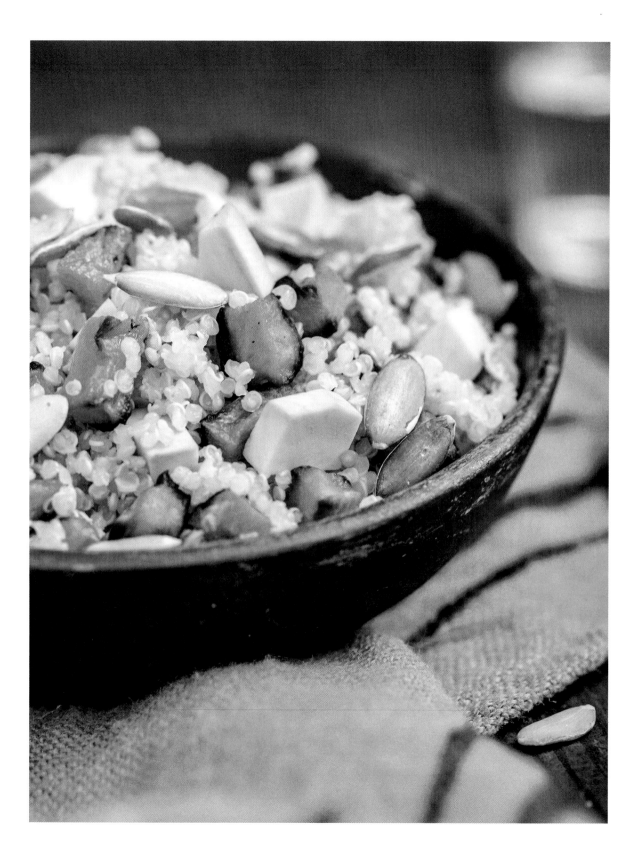

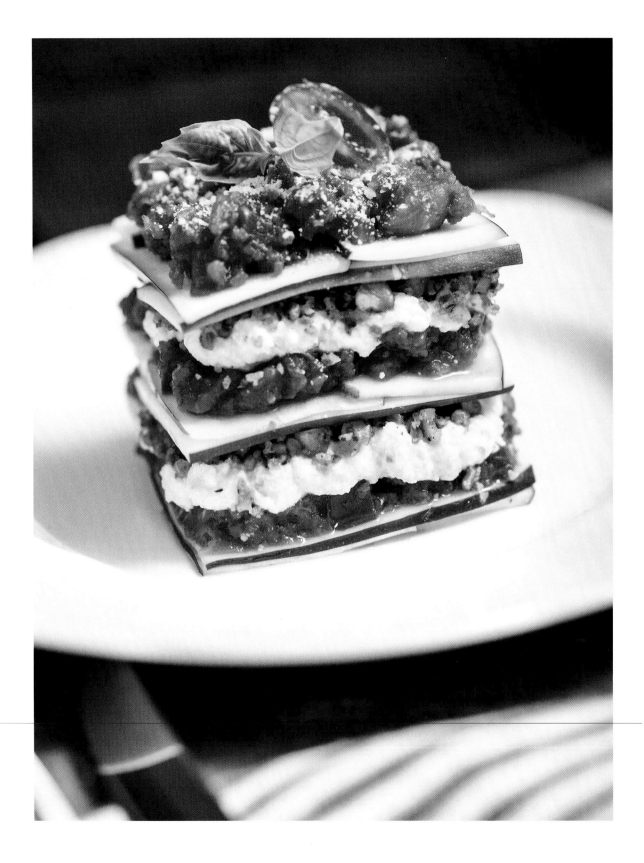

RAW LASAGNA

PREP TIME: 40 min

COOK TIME: 0 min

TOTAL TIME: 40 min

MAKES 4 SERVINGS

Health is not usually not the first thing you think of when you see lasagna. Well, we're about to change that. This lasagna is completely raw and full of vitamins, minerals, and powerful phytochemicals for a guilt-free trip to Italy.

INGREDIENTS FOR TOMATO SAUCE (MAKES ABOUT ¾–1 CUP):

1 large tomato

¼ cup sun-dried tomatoes

4 fresh basil leaves

pinch of dried oregano

pinch of sea salt

INGREDIENTS FOR LASAGNA:

¾ cup Cashew Cheese (see recipe on page 320) (about 12 tablespoons)

½ cup Walnut Meat (see recipe on page 347) (about 8 tablespoons)

4 tablespoons Parmesan Cheese or to taste (see recipe on page 340)

4 large zucchini, washed and ends trimmed

4 cherry tomatoes, washed and halved, for garnish

basil leaves, for garnish

ground black pepper, to taste

PREPARATION:

1. To prepare the tomato sauce, combine all the ingredients in a food processor and blend until smooth. Refrigerate the sauce in an air-tight container until ready to use.

2. Prepare the Cashew Cheese, the Walnut Meat, and Parmesan Cheese according to their recipes and store them in the refrigerator until ready to use.

3. Use a mandolin or vegetable peeler to cut the zucchini in thin slices, lengthwise. Then cut the slices in half.

4. To make 4 individual stacks: On each serving plate, place a layer of 3–4 zucchini slices, slightly overlapping them. Top with about 1½ tablespoons of tomato sauce, then 1½ tablespoons of Cashew Cheese, then 2 tablespoons of Walnut Meat. Add another layer of zucchini slices, arranged in the opposite direction from the first layer. Top with 1½ tablespoons of tomato sauce, then 1½ tablespoons of Cashew Cheese. Make another layer of zucchini slices (in the opposite direction of the previous layer), topped with 1½ tablespoons of tomato sauce. Sprinkle with Parmesan Cheese and garnish with cherry tomatoes and basil. Season with freshly ground black pepper and serve.

Recipe continues

VARIATION:

▸ To prepare the lasagna in one baking dish, line the base with a layer of zucchini slices, slightly overlapping them. Then add layers of tomato sauce, Cashew Cheese, and Walnut Meat. Repeat with additional layers of zucchini slices, tomato sauce, and Cashew Cheese, followed by a final layer of zucchini slices and tomato sauce. Sprinkle with Parmesan Cheese; garnish with cherry tomatoes and basil. Season with freshly ground black pepper.

NOTE: The lasagna is best if refrigerated for a few hours so that it can harden slightly, making it a little easier to cut into portions. Keep refrigerated until ready to serve! Best if enjoyed within a day or two.

PER SERVING: 286 calories, 12 grams protein, 26 grams carbohydrates, 18 grams total fat

INDULGENT MEALS

(300 CALORIES OR MORE)

It may seem counterintuitive, but it's not! Plant-based, vegan meals can be nutrient-dense *and* indulgent. The flavors and textures in these recipes have been developed to satisfy big appetites and picky eaters, while packing a mega-veggie punch. Our comfort foods are so tasty and hearty that your friends might not believe they're good for you! These recipes are the trusted and favorite classics that you and your family have reached to for decades. Our take on these favorites lightens them up, providing that satisfying and familiar flavor you love in a new and healthy way.

It is possible to create meals that are delicious period, not just delicious for "vegan food." And these recipes are proof that it's absolutely possible, and your body will thank you!

INDULGENT

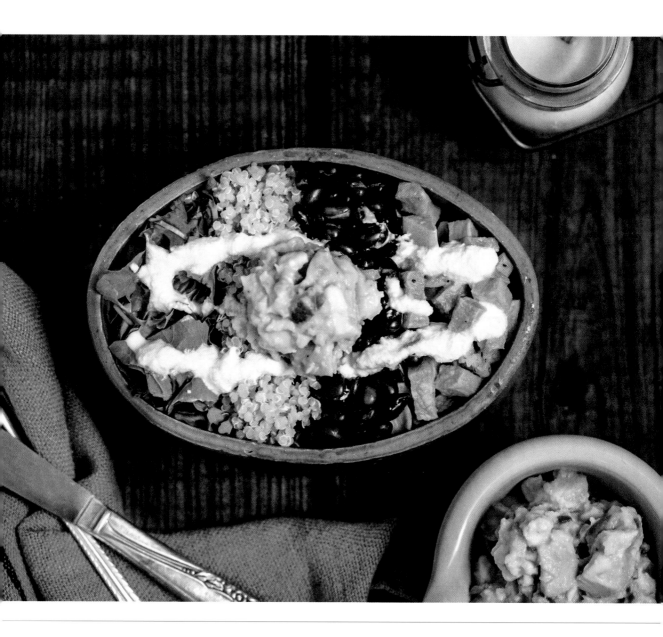

BLACK BEAN, SWEET POTATO & QUINOA SALAD

PREP TIME: 15 min

COOK TIME: 55 min

TOTAL TIME: 70 min (does not include Black Beans cook time)

MAKES 4 SERVINGS

This is a dish that was inspired by my Cuban roots. When I was growing up, we ate tons of white rice and black beans, and I loved them. Here, we've created a healthier version loaded with vitamins, minerals, and phytochemicals for a nostalgic dish that nourishes the mind and body.

INGREDIENTS:

3 cups cooked Quinoa (see recipe on page 343)

1½ cups cooked Black Beans (see recipe on page 315) or 1 15-ounce can, rinsed and drained

1 large sweet potato, diced into small cubes

sea salt, to taste

ground black pepper, to taste

Guacamole (see recipe on page 246)

1 5-ounce package of baby arugula

¼ cup pumpkin seeds (pepitas)

Cashew Cream Dressing (see recipe on page 323)

PREPARATION:

1. Preheat oven to 400F and line a baking sheet with parchment paper.

2. If you prepared the quinoa and black beans fresh for this recipe, set them aside to cool.

3. Spread the sweet potatoes on the baking sheet with a pinch of sea salt and pepper.

4. Bake for about 30 minutes, tossing occasionally, until soft and golden.

5. Meanwhile, prepare the guacamole.

6. Prepare a serving dish, or 4 individual bowls, by layering first with the arugula, then the quinoa, the black beans, the sweet potatoes, and guacamole.

7. Top with pumpkin seeds and a drizzle of dressing, and enjoy!

TIP: Leftovers can be stored for up to 4 days, but guacamole is best if stored separately, and for no more than 1 day.

PER SERVING: 363 calories, 17 grams protein, 58 grams carbohydrates, 9 grams total fat

FENNEL & ARUGULA SALAD WITH AVOCADO, CHICKPEAS, AND PARMESAN

PREP TIME: 15 min

COOK TIME: 0 min

TOTAL TIME: 15 min

MAKES 4 SERVINGS

Fennel has a very unique taste, and when paired correctly, it can be phenomenally tasty. Here's a great pairing of nutrients and flavor.

INGREDIENTS:

1 fennel bulb

4 radishes, washed

2 tablespoons extra-virgin olive oil

1 lime, juiced

½ teaspoon sea salt, or to taste

ground black pepper, to taste

1 15-ounce can chickpeas

3 cups arugula, tightly packed, washed, and drained

1 Hass avocado, halved, cored, peeled, and chopped

Parmesan Cheese (see recipe on page 340)

PREPARATION:

1. To prepare the fennel, remove the stalks and fronds by cutting as close to the bulb as possible. Cut the bulb in half from top to bottom and then remove the core.

2. To prepare the washed radishes, trim the ends.

3. Using a mandolin slicer, thinly shave the fennel bulb and the radishes and transfer the slices to a mixing bowl.

4. Toss the fennel and radishes with the oil, lime, salt, and pepper; set aside so that the flavors settle in.

5. To prepare the chickpeas, drain and rinse, discarding some of the thin skin.

6. Gently toss the chickpeas, arugula, and avocado together with the fennel and radish. Taste and adjust seasoning, if necessary.

7. Serve on a platter or on 4 individual plates with a sprinkling of Parmesan Cheese and enjoy!

NOTE: Image shown with walnuts.

PER SERVING: 312 calories, 8 grams protein, 26 grams carbohydrates, 22 grams total fat

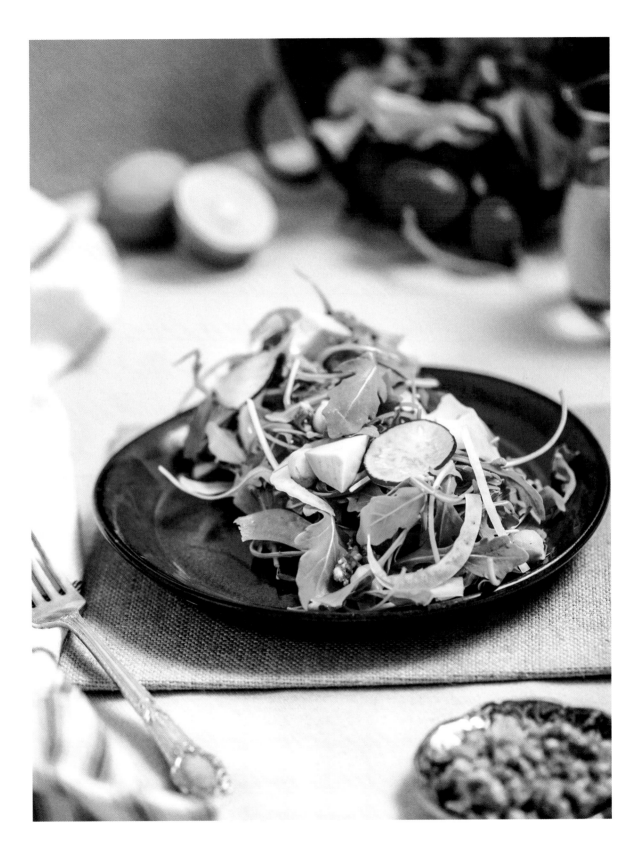

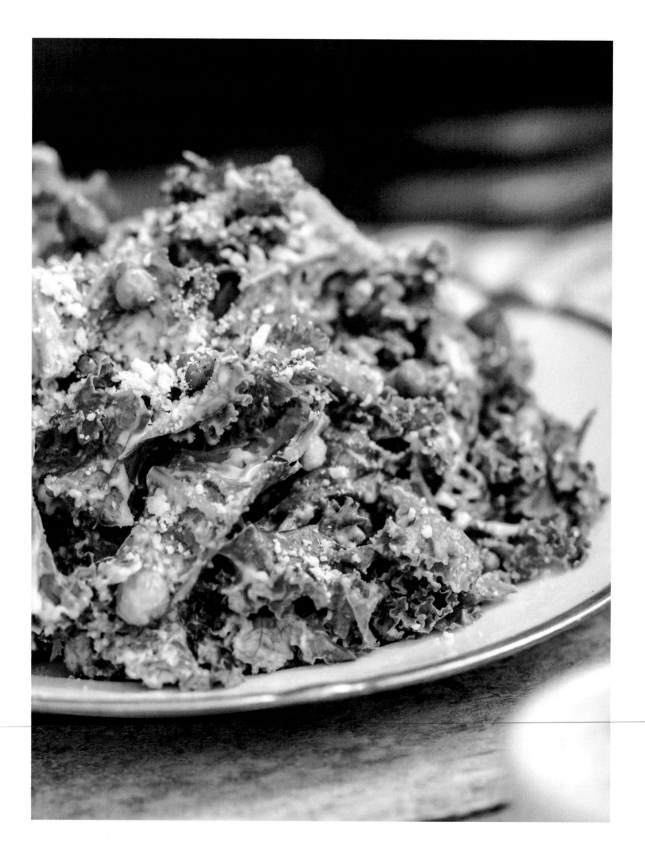

KALE CAESAR SALAD

PREP TIME: 20 min

COOK TIME: 0 min

TOTAL TIME: 20 min

MAKES 2 SERVINGS

Did you give up dairy and now miss Caesar salads? Problem solved. This recipe is quite simple and better than the real thing. Serve it at your next family dinner, and watch as they all enjoy in disbelief.

INGREDIENTS:

Crunchy Chickpeas (see recipe on page 242)

Parmesan Cheese (see recipe on page 340), to taste

Caesar Dressing (see recipe below)

2 5-ounce packages baby kale

FOR CAESAR DRESSING:

½ cup raw cashews

¼ cup water, adding 1 more tablespoon at a time if necessary

1 tablespoon nutritional yeast

2 tablespoons lemon juice

½ tablespoon Dijon mustard

1 small garlic clove or ½ teaspoon garlic powder

½ teaspoon sea salt

PREPARATION:

1. First prepare the Crunchy Chickpeas and Parmesan Cheese. Set aside.

2. To prepare the Caesar Dressing, presoak the cashews for 30 minutes in hot water. Drain and rinse the cashews, then add all dressing ingredients to a high-speed blender (or food processor) and blend until the dressing is creamy and smooth.

3. To prepare the salad, thoroughly wash and dry the kale in a colander. In a large mixing bowl, toss the kale together with the Caesar Dressing, making sure to coat all leaves. Serve and top with Crunchy Chickpeas and Parmesan Cheese, and enjoy!

NOTE: The preparation time doesn't include the cashews soaking time.

VARIATION:

▶ The baby kale can be substituted for chopped lacinato kale and/or romaine lettuce.

PER SERVING: 454 calories, 20 grams protein, 40 grams carbohydrates, 28 grams total fat

LENTIL & KALE SALAD WITH ARTICHOKE HEARTS & SUN-DRIED TOMATOES

PREP TIME: 30 min

COOK TIME: 30 min

TOTAL TIME: 60 min

MAKES 4 SERVINGS

Lentils are a wonderful protein source and one of very few protein sources that are alkaline, which means they reduce acidity in the body. I love the blend of textures this dish offers in an explosion of flavors that will keep you going back for more.

INGREDIENTS:

1 cup uncooked French green lentils or other lentils

3 cups water

pinch salt

5 cups finely chopped curly kale, thoroughly washed and destemmed

3 cups finely chopped romaine lettuce

1 Hass avocado, halved, pitted, peeled, and sliced into cubes

½ small onion, thinly sliced

¼ cup sun-dried tomatoes, thinly sliced

4 canned artichoke hearts, drained and quartered

2 lemons, juiced

2 tablespoons extra-virgin olive oil

¼ teaspoon sea salt or to taste

pine nuts, for garnish, to taste

PREPARATION:

1. To prepare the lentils, rinse them in a colander while discarding any stones.

2. In a medium pot over high heat, add the lentils, water, and a pinch of salt, and bring to a boil.

3. Reduce the heat to a simmer, partially cover the pot, and cook for about 25–30 minutes or until tender. Drain and let the lentils cool until ready to use.

4. In a mixing bowl, add the lentils, kale, romaine lettuce, avocados, onions, sun-dried tomatoes, and artichoke hearts and gently toss to combine.

5. Add the lemon juice, oil, and sea salt and toss once more.

6. Transfer the salad to a serving bowl, garnish with pine nuts, and enjoy!

PER SERVING: 409 calories, 20 grams protein, 50 grams carbohydrates, 18 grams total fat

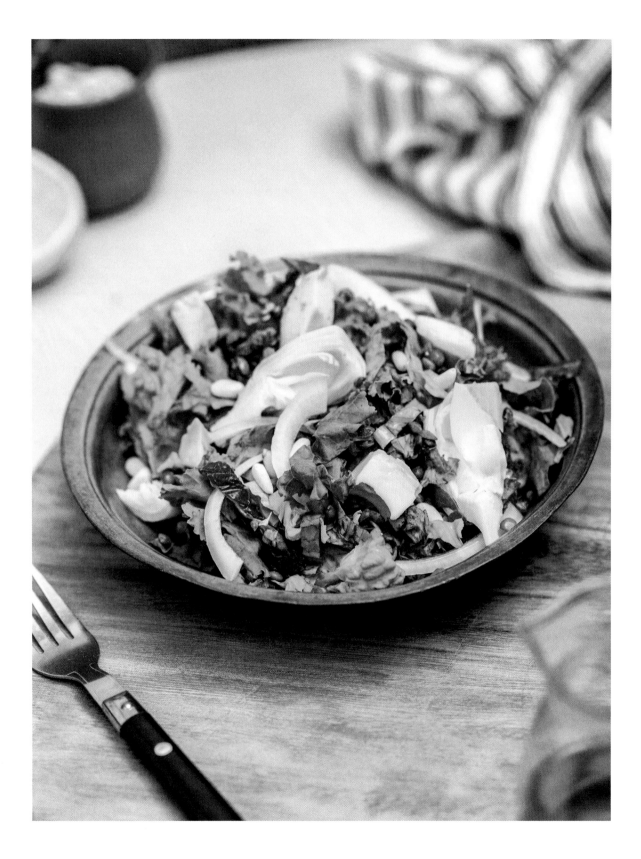

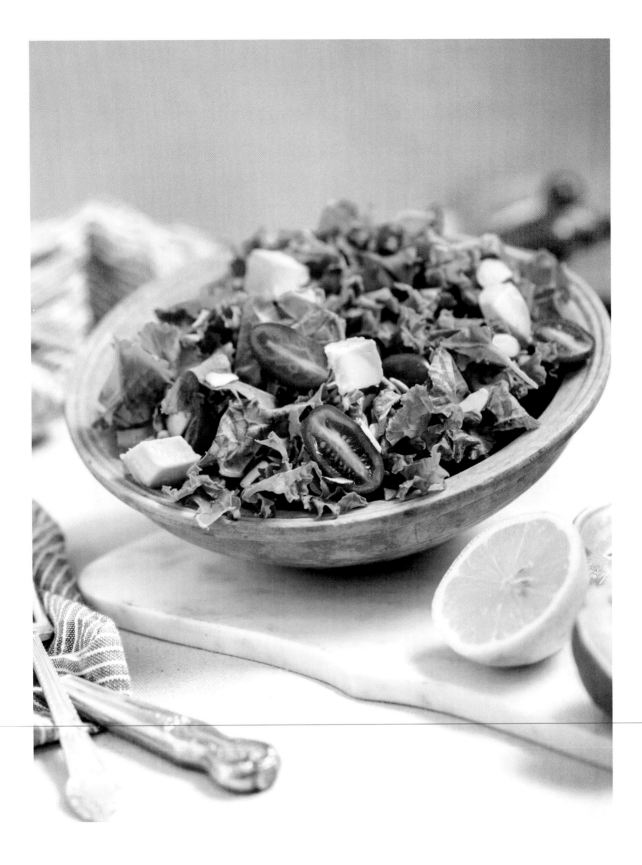

RAW KALE & AVOCADO SALAD

PREP TIME: 15 min

COOK TIME: 0 min

TOTAL TIME: 15 min

MAKES 2 SERVINGS

This can easily become a go-to favorite in any home for its nutrient density and delicious flavors. Enjoy it at any time of the day or night.

INGREDIENTS:

dressing (see recipe below)

4 cups chopped kale

1 small Hass avocado

½ cup grape tomatoes

2 tablespoons sunflower seeds

2 tablespoons almonds, sliced

INGREDIENTS FOR DRESSING:

4 tablespoons lemon juice

1 tablespoon extra-virgin olive oil

pinch of fresh pepper

sea salt, to taste

PREPARATION:

1. Make the dressing by whisking together all dressing ingredients. Taste and adjust the seasonings for desired flavor.

2. Toss the kale into a mixing bowl and add the dressing. Gently massage the dressing into the kale to soften.

3. Cut the avocado into small cubes and slice the tomatoes.

4. Add the rest of the ingredients to the mixing bowl, lightly toss together and enjoy.

PER SERVING: 407 calories, 12 grams protein, 30 grams carbohydrates, 31 grams total fat

SWEET BROCCOLI SALAD WITH MICRO-GREENS

PREP TIME: 15 min
COOK TIME: 5 min
TOTAL TIME: 20 min

MAKES 1 SERVING

We all know we should be eating more greens (vegetables) but often find ourselves wondering how to make them more exciting and tasty. This dish is quick and easy, and it is yet another fun way to eat more greens. The whole family will enjoy this one!

INGREDIENTS:

1 cup broccoli florets

1 cup microgreens

½ cup alfalfa sprouts

dressing (see recipe below)

¼ cup raw almonds, sliced

INGREDIENTS FOR DRESSING:

2 tablespoons balsamic vinegar

1 tablespoon lemon juice

2 teaspoons maple syrup

½ teaspoon ground cumin

½ teaspoon smoked paprika

PREPARATION:

1. Steam the broccoli for 4–5 minutes until bright green.

2. Chop the broccoli and toss it into a large mixing bowl with the microgreens and alfalfa sprouts.

3. In a separate small bowl, whisk together all the dressing ingredients.

4. Serve the broccoli salad topped with sliced almonds and a drizzle of dressing, to taste.

PER SERVING: 345 calories, 9 grams protein, 52 grams carbohydrates, 12 grams total fat

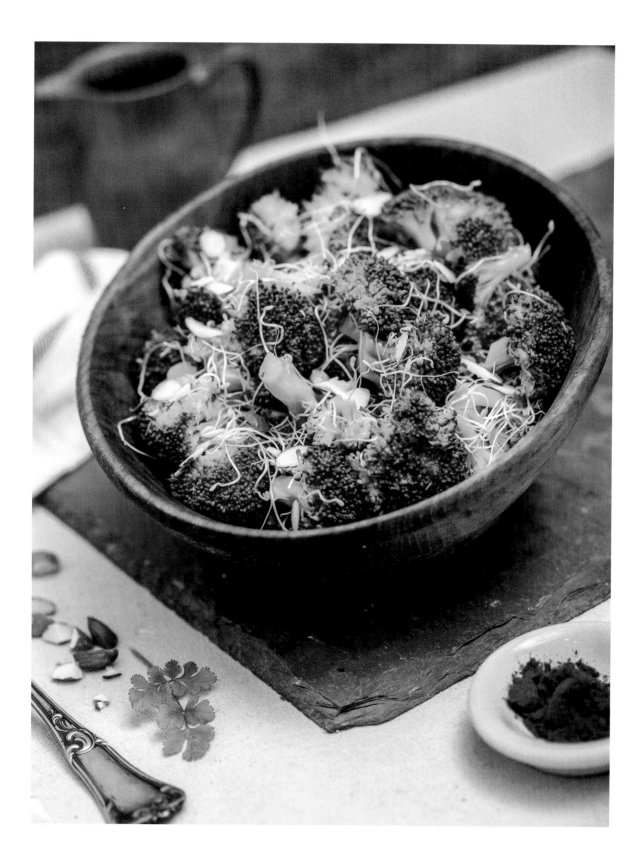

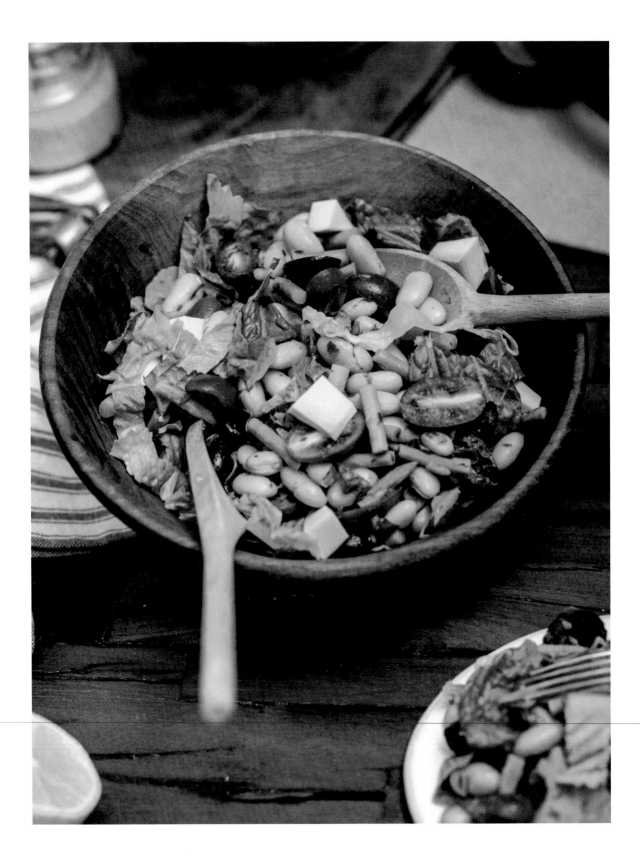

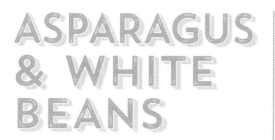

ASPARAGUS & WHITE BEANS

PREP TIME: 20 min

COOK TIME: 3 min

TOTAL TIME: 23 min

MAKES 4 SERVINGS

Asparagus is loaded with fiber, folate, chromium, and vitamins A, C, E, and K. Consider the protein, folate, and antioxidant and detox properties from the white beans a freebie.

INGREDIENTS:

8 asparagus stalks, trimmed and sliced into ½-inch to 1-inch pieces

2 15-ounce cans cannellini beans (unsalted), drained and rinsed

2 cups thinly sliced romaine lettuce

¼ cup parsley flakes

1 cup cherry tomatoes, halved

¼ cup Kalamata olives, pitted and sliced

Lemon Dijon Vinaigrette Dressing (see recipe on page 335), to taste

1 Hass avocado, halved, cored, peeled, and sliced into cubes

PREPARATION:

1. In a small pot of salted water, boil the asparagus for 2–3 minutes. Drain and rinse with cold water.

2. In a large mixing bowl, combine the asparagus, beans, romaine lettuce, parsley, tomatoes, and olives.

3. Prepare the dressing and toss together. Then fold in the avocados and gently combine.

4. Transfer the salad to a serving bowl and enjoy!

PER SERVING: 341 calories, 16 grams protein, 42 grams carbohydrates, 14 grams total fat

INDULGENT

HEARTS OF PALM & CANNELLINI

PREP TIME: 20 min

COOK TIME: 0 min

TOTAL TIME: 20 min

MAKES 2 SERVINGS

Hearts of palm are loaded with potassium, which helps regulate our heartbeat and lowers blood pressure and is rich in B_6. Cannellini beans are a great source of complex carbs and protein as well as B vitamins, iron, zinc, and minerals, which makes this easy-to-make salad a favorite among athletes.

INGREDIENTS:

1 14-ounce can hearts of palm

1 15-ounce can cannellini beans (unsalted), drained and rinsed

1 cup cherry tomatoes, halved

½ cup finely sliced curly kale or leafy green of choice, thoroughly washed and destemmed

½ small red onion, thinly sliced

1 tablespoon extra-virgin olive oil, to taste

1 lime, juiced

¼ teaspoon sea salt or to taste

ground black pepper, to taste

PREPARATION:

1. To prepare the hearts of palm, drain in a colander and slice into ½-inch-thick pieces. Transfer into a mixing bowl, and separate some pieces into rings.

2. To the bowl, add the cannellini beans, tomatoes, kale, and red onion.

3. Toss together with extra-virgin olive oil, lime juice, sea salt, and pepper. Serve and enjoy.

PER SERVING: 334 calories, 19 grams protein, 51 grams carbohydrates, 9 grams total fat

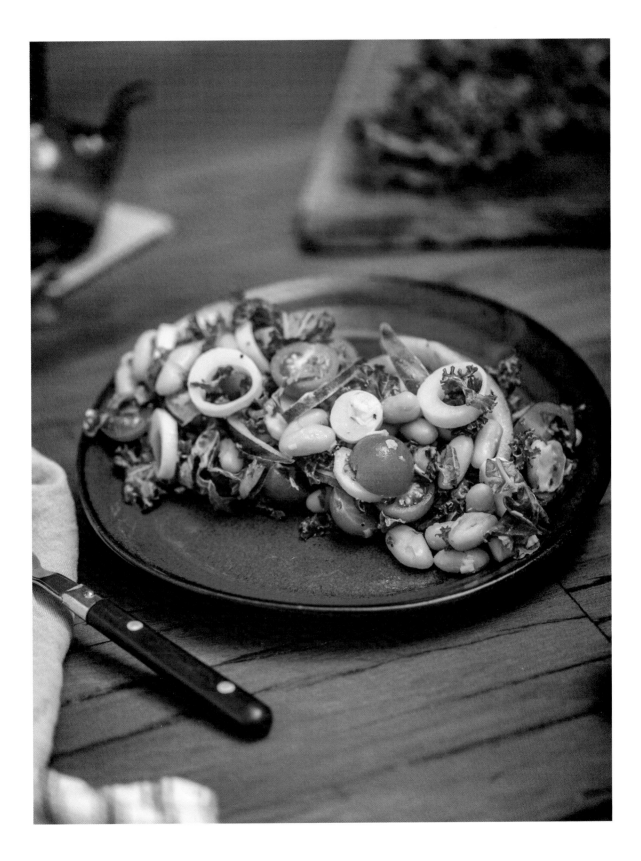

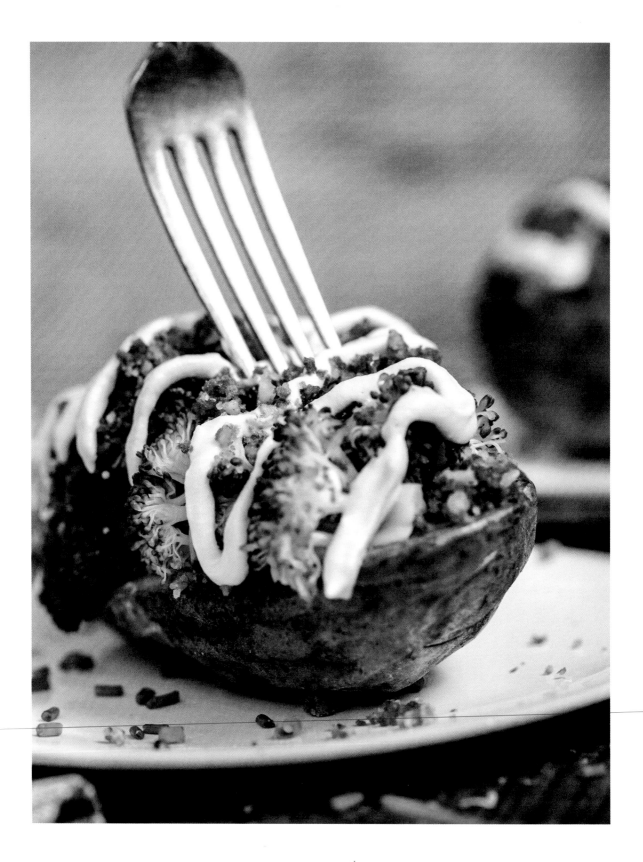

LOADED BAKED POTATO

PREP TIME: 20 min

COOK TIME: 45 min

TOTAL TIME: 65 min

MAKES 2 SERVINGS

Potatoes are a rich source of vitamin C, B_6, magnesium, iron, and calcium. The walnuts add heart-healthy omega-3 fatty acids, and the broccoli adds in some cancer protection and anti-inflammatory properties, which all add up to an incredibly powerful dish you no longer have to pass on.

Feel free to substitute the russet (or Yukon gold) potatoes with sweet potatoes. Either works well in this recipe and is just as delicious.

INGREDIENTS:

canola oil or oil of choice, for coating

2 large russet or Yukon gold potatoes

sea salt, to taste

Cashew Cheese (see recipe on page 320), to taste

½ cup Walnut Meat (see recipe on page 347)

2 cups small broccoli florets

chives, finely chopped, for garnish

PREPARATION:

1. Preheat oven to 400F and lightly grease a baking sheet with oil of choice or line with parchment paper.

2. Scrub and rinse the potatoes. Slice them in half, lengthwise. Poke with a fork a couple times and lightly coat with oil and a pinch of sea salt.

3. Place potatoes facedown on the baking sheet, and bake for about 35–45 minutes or until the potatoes are fork tender.

4. Meanwhile, prepare the Cashew Cheese and Walnut Meat according to their recipes and set aside until ready to use. Store leftovers as suggested in recipe.

5. Wash the broccoli and place it in a steaming basket over a pot of boiling water. Reduce the heat, add a pinch of salt, cover, and steam for 6–8 minutes or until desired tenderness is reached.

6. When the potatoes are tender, place them in a serving dish with flesh up and poke a couple times with a fork to slightly mash and open the flesh.

7. Top the potatoes with broccoli florets and Walnut Meat, sprinkle with Cashew Cheese, garnish with chives, and enjoy.

PER SERVING: 485 calories, 14 grams protein, 76 grams carbohydrates, 16 grams total fat

ENDIVE SALAD CUPS

PREP TIME: 25 min

COOK TIME: 0 min

TOTAL TIME: 25 min (does not include Black Beans cook time)

MAKES 4 SERVINGS

These salad cups are as fun and as light as they look. They're a crowd-pleaser and perfect for parties. Loaded with vitamins A, K, B$_1$, B$_3$, B$_5$, and B$_6$, they're as beneficial for our health as they are for our reputations as a host.

INGREDIENTS:

4 heads Belgian endive (about 24 leaves)

1 15-ounce can chickpeas

1½ cups cooked Black Beans (see recipe on page 315) or 1 15-ounce can

1 cup cherry tomatoes, halved or quartered

1 cup fresh parsley, chopped

1 small red pepper, seeded and diced

1 small green pepper, seeded and diced

¼ cup diced onion

1 Hass avocado, halved, cored, peeled, and chopped

dash garlic powder

dash ground black pepper

Balsamic Vinaigrette Dressing (see recipe on page 311) or Lemon Dijon Vinaigrette Dressing (see recipe on page 335)

PREPARATION:

1. Separate the endive leaves, then wash and dry them in a colander. Select the 24 largest leaves for use as your cups.

2. Thinly slice the remaining smaller leaves and transfer them to a mixing bowl.

3. Add the chickpeas, black beans, tomatoes, parsley, peppers, onions, and avocados and gently toss together with the dressing of choice.

4. Top each endive leaf with the salad mixture, garnish with parsley, and serve!

PER SERVING: 430 calories, 20 grams protein, 61 grams carbohydrates, 15 grams total fat

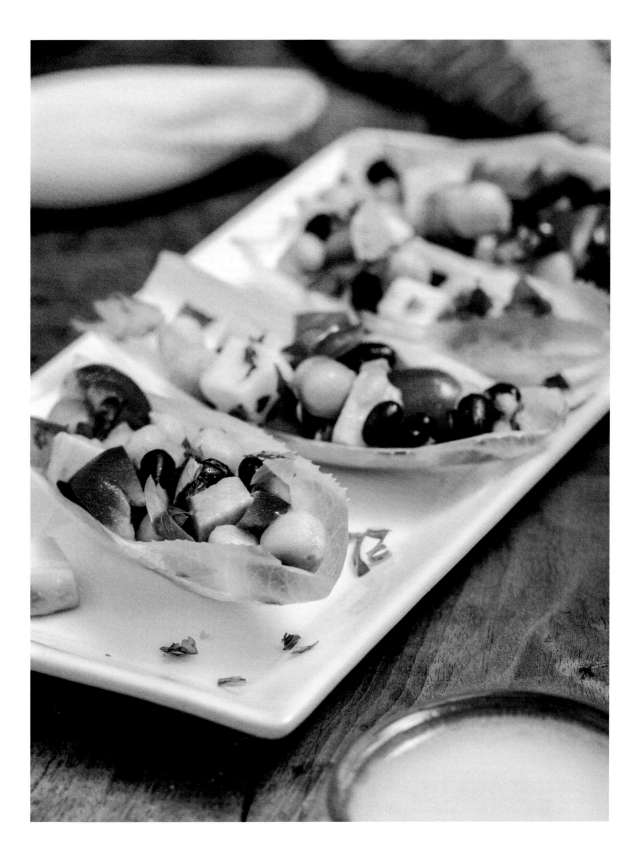

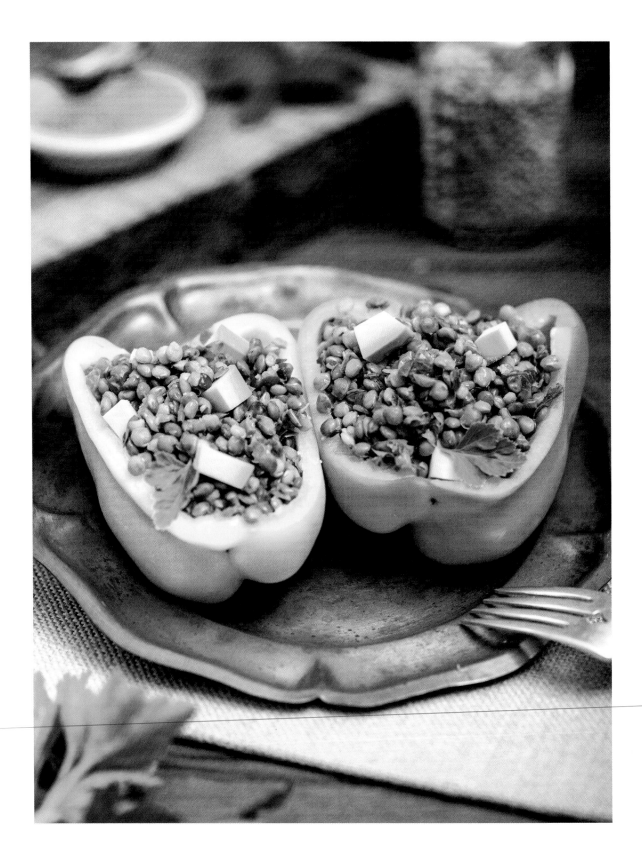

STUFFED BELL PEPPER CUPS WITH LENTILS & AVOCADO

PREP TIME: 15 min

COOK TIME: 30 min

TOTAL TIME: 45 min

MAKES 4 SERVINGS

Bell peppers are low in calories and high in nutrition! They're loaded with vitamin C, phytochemicals, and carotenoids for a healthy immune system. These are stuffed with one of our favorite protein sources and topped with avocados, which contain heart-healthy omega-3 fatty acids.

INGREDIENTS:

1½ cups dry green or brown lentils (about 4½ cups cooked)

1 tablespoon canola oil or oil of choice

½ onion, finely chopped

¼ teaspoon garlic, minced

½ teaspoon sea salt or to taste

5 cups water

½ teaspoon cumin

½ teaspoon coriander

¼ teaspoon turmeric

dash cayenne pepper

2 Hass avocados, halved, cored, and chopped

1 lime, juiced

½ teaspoon parsley, minced

dash sea salt

4 large bell peppers (red, yellow, or green), washed, halved lengthwise (to form cups), and seeded

Lemon Dijon Vinaigrette Dressing (see recipe on page 335) or Creamy Cashew Balsamic Vinaigrette Dressing (see recipe on page 327)

PREPARATION:

1. To prepare the lentils, sift through them and remove any tiny stones you find. Rinse lentils well in a colander.

2. In a saucepan, heat the canola oil over medium-high heat. Add the onions, garlic, and a dash of salt, stirring occasionally until the onions become translucent.

3. Add the sorted and rinsed lentils, water, cumin, coriander, turmeric, and cayenne, and bring to a boil.

4. Reduce to a simmer, cover, and cook for about 30 minutes, stirring occasionally to avoid burning or sticking to the pot.

Recipe continues

5. Once the lentils are tender, remove the saucepan from the stove and rinse the lentils with cool water. Set them aside to cool completely while preparing the other ingredients.

6. In a mixing bowl, add the avocados, lime juice, parsley, salt, and lentils and lightly toss together.

7. Scoop the salad into the pepper halves, drizzle with dressing, and serve!

TIP: Leftovers can be stored in the refrigerator for up to 4–5 days. This recipe is also delicious if topped with Pico de Gallo (see recipe on page 249).

PER SERVING WITH 2 TABLESPOONS LEMON DIJON VINAIGRETTE DRESSING : 478 calories, 22 grams protein, 63 grams carbohydrates, 17 grams total fat

BBQ MEATLESS BALL SKEWERS

PREP TIME: 25 min

COOK TIME: 75 min

TOTAL TIME: 100 min

MAKES 2 SERVINGS

Sometimes it's not so much the meat that people miss when they move toward a plant-based diet but rather the experience of certain foods. For example, I noticed that I didn't really miss sushi when I went plant-based but rather the "eating with chop sticks and dipping in sauces" part of the experience. So I opted for veggie rolls and began making sauces at home. BBQ is another one of these experiences. These meatless ball skewers are incredibly tasty and satisfy all the senses that crave BBQ without the meat.

INGREDIENTS:

1 tablespoon canola oil, for skillet

2 cups sliced white mushrooms, washed

1 small onion, diced (about ½ cup)

1 garlic clove, minced

1 teaspoon sea salt or to taste

½ teaspoon ground cumin

1½ cups cooked Short-Grain Brown Rice (see recipe on page 319)

3 tablespoons gluten-free flour (brown rice flour)

¼ cup plus 2 tablespoons gluten-free bread crumbs (reserve ¼ cup for coating)

½ teaspoon dried parsley

½ teaspoon dried basil

¼ teaspoon ground black pepper or to taste

⅛ teaspoon dried oregano

FOR THE SKEWERS:

1 large red pepper, cut into bite-size pieces

1 large green pepper, cut into bite-size pieces

1 small onion, cut into bite-size pieces

BBQ Sauce (see recipe on page 312)

PREPARATION:

1. Preheat oven to 400F. Line a baking sheet with parchment paper.

2. Heat the canola oil in a large skillet over medium-high heat and sauté the mushrooms, onions, garlic, dash of salt, and cumin until the mushrooms and onions are soft. Set aside to cool.

3. In a food processor, add the mushroom mixture with the brown rice, gluten-free flour, 2 tablespoons of gluten-free bread crumbs, parsley, basil, pepper, and oregano and pulse until well combined.

Recipe continues

4. Using your hands, form about 18–22 table-spoon-sized meatballs. Coat the meatballs with remaining bread crumbs.

5. To each long skewer stick, add the peppers, onions, and meatless meatballs (3–4 to a skewer), repeating the ingredients to create a pattern.

6. Lightly brush skewered ingredients with BBQ Sauce and bake for 18–20 minutes, rotating once or twice for even browning.

7. Serve the skewers with extra BBQ Sauce for dipping and enjoy! These can be enjoyed simply or with a mixed green salad.

PER SERVING WITH 2 TABLESPOONS BBQ SAUCE:
409 calories, 10 grams protein, 75 grams carbohydrates, 10 grams total fat

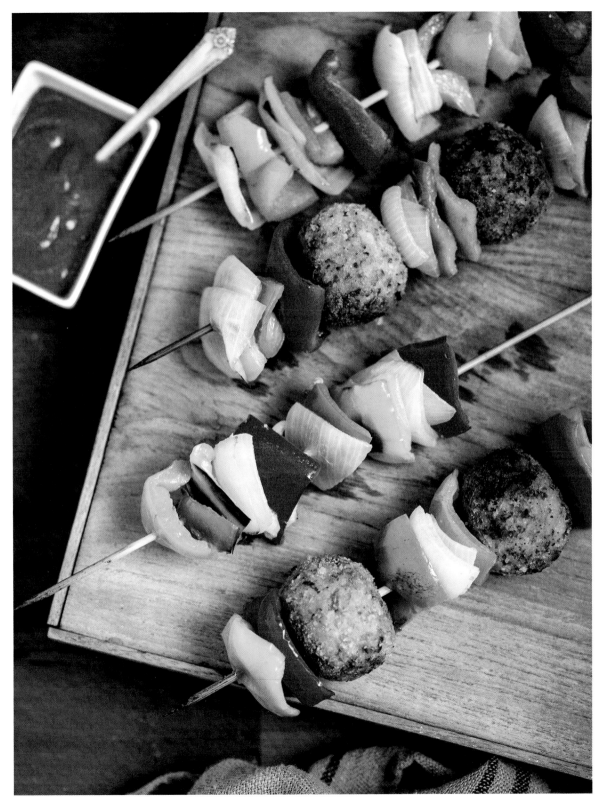

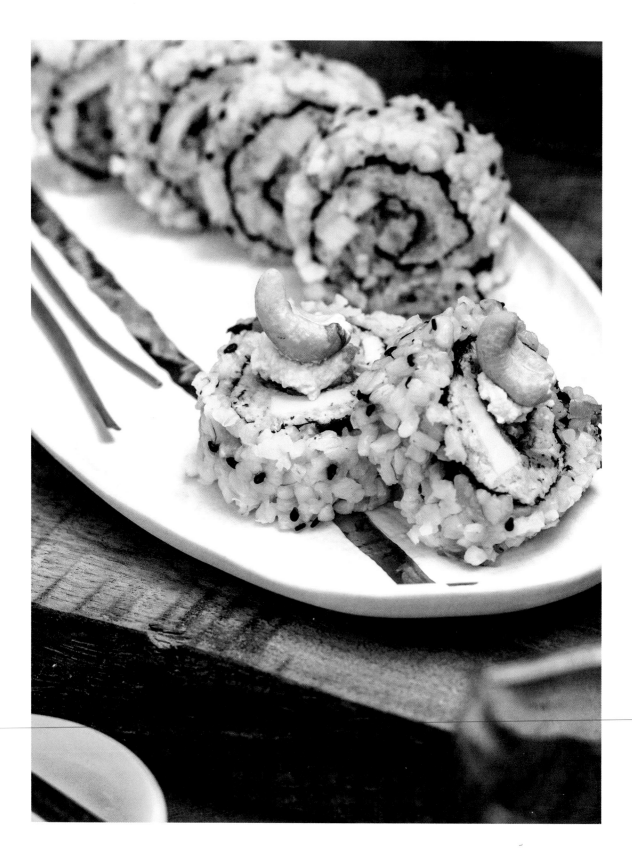

CASHEW CHICKPEA SUSHI ROLL

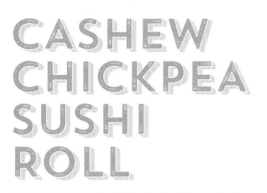

PREP TIME: 25 min

COOK TIME: 55 min

TOTAL TIME: 80 min (time includes Short-Grain Brown Rice but does not include Cashew Cheese recipe)

MAKES 1 SERVING

Making sushi is fun and easy, once you get the hang of it. The first few times, it might not look so pretty, but don't get discouraged. Give it a try!

This recipe makes 1 serving. Feel free to double the recipe for more servings.

INGREDIENTS FOR SUSHI:

1 cup cooked Short-Grain Brown Rice (see recipe on page 319)

1 tablespoon brown rice vinegar

½ cup cooked chickpeas

2–3 tablespoons Cashew Cheese (see recipe on page 320) or the mayo of choice, plus extra for topping

1 nori sheet

1 tablespoon sesame seeds

¼ Hass avocado, peeled, pitted, and thinly sliced

1 small carrot, finely shredded (about ¼ cup)

6–8 cashews, roasted and salted

coconut aminos (soy-sauce alternative) or other sauce of choice, for serving

2 tablespoons diced scallions

SUPPLIES:

bamboo rolling mat

plastic wrap

PREPARATION:

1. Place 1 cup of cooked rice in a large bowl and mix with 1 tablespoon of brown rice vinegar. Set aside and let it reach room temperature.

2. To prepare the chickpea "tuna," rinse and drain the chickpeas, then transfer them to a food processor along with the Cashew Cheese.

3. Pulse a few times until well combined.

4. To prepare the sushi roll, completely cover the bamboo mat with plastic wrap and set aside.

5. Place the nori with the rough side facing upward (shiny side down).

6. Wet your hands to prevent the rice from sticking to your fingers. Place the brown rice in the middle of the nori.

7. Evenly spread the rice with your fingers while pressing down gently. Sprinkle the sesame seeds over the rice.

8. Flip the nori over and place it on top of the bamboo mat.

Recipe continues

9. Spread the chickpea tuna across the middle of the nori. Add the avocados and carrots.

10. Use the bamboo mat to roll the bottom edge of the nori over the filling, keeping it tight and applying pressure with every move forward. Press and smooth the ends.

11. Remove the roll from the mat. With a sharp knife, cut the nori into 6–8 pieces.

12. Flip each piece sideways with filling facing upward and top each piece with about ¼–½ teaspoon of Cashew Cheese and one cashew.

13. To prepare the dipping sauce, pour the coconut aminos and scallions into a small bowl and enjoy!

PER SERVING: 558 calories, 17 grams protein, 88 grams carbohydrates, 20 grams total fat

FALAFEL BOWL

PREP TIME: 20 min

COOK TIME: 10 min

TOTAL TIME: 30 min

MAKES 4 SERVINGS

We love baked falafel topped with our favorite Tahini Dressing. It adds an exciting and delicious crunch to salads and bowls or can be enjoyed alone.

FOR THE FALAFEL:

¾ cup chopped curly parsley

½ cup chopped scallions

2 cloves garlic

6 tablespoons lemon juice

2 15-ounce cans chickpeas, drained and rinsed, reserving ¼ cup of the liquid (3 cups cooked)

½ cup gluten-free chickpea flour or gluten-free oat flour

1 tablespoon ground cumin

1 teaspoon ground turmeric

1 teaspoon coriander

1 teaspoon paprika

dash of ground black pepper

sea salt, to taste

FOR THE KALE SALAD:

1 bunch lacinato or curly kale, washed, de-stemmed and finely chopped (about 4 cups)

½ small head of romaine, washed and chopped (about 2 cups)

1 Hass avocado, halved, cored, peeled, and sliced

2 small carrots, shredded

2 small cucumbers, sliced

4 radishes, sliced

1 red pepper, sliced

1 cup cherry tomatoes, washed and halved

Kalamata olives, sliced

Tahini Dressing (see recipe on page 344)

PREPARATION:

1. To make the falafel, pulse the parsley, scallions, and garlic in a food processor. Add the lemon juice and blend.

2. Add the remaining ingredients and pulse until well combined. Use a spoon to help scrape down the mixture from the sides. If the mixture is too dry, add the chickpea water as needed to loosen it.

3. Form the dough into 8 small patties and place them on a lightly greased skillet over medium-high heat for about 4–5 minutes. Flip the patties and cook for another 5 minutes until the patties are golden brown.

4. If you prefer to bake the falafel, preheat oven to 375F. Grease a baking sheet with oil of choice or line with parchment paper, and bake the patties for 15–20 minutes. Flip the patties and bake them for another 10 minutes or until golden brown.

Recipe continues

5. To prepare the kale salad, divide the kale and romaine into 4 bowls. Then layer in the sliced avocados, carrots, cucumbers, radishes, peppers, cherry tomatoes, and olives. Top each bowl with 2 falafel patties and drizzle with Tahini Dressing and serve!

TIP: Leftover patties can be stored in refrigerator for up to a week or in freezer for a few months.

PER SERVING WITH 2 TABLESPOONS OF DRESSING: 376 calories, 17 grams protein, 54 grams carbohydrates, 13 grams total fat

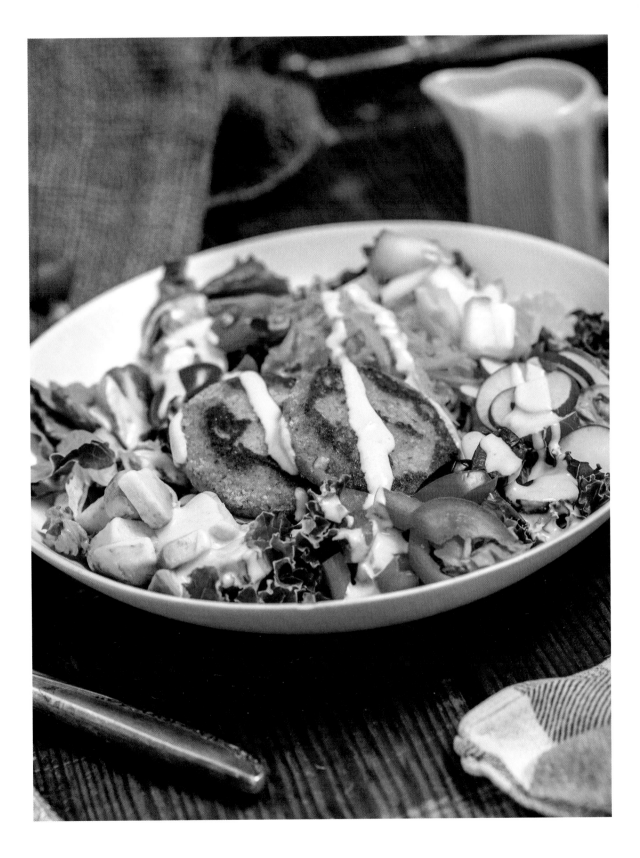

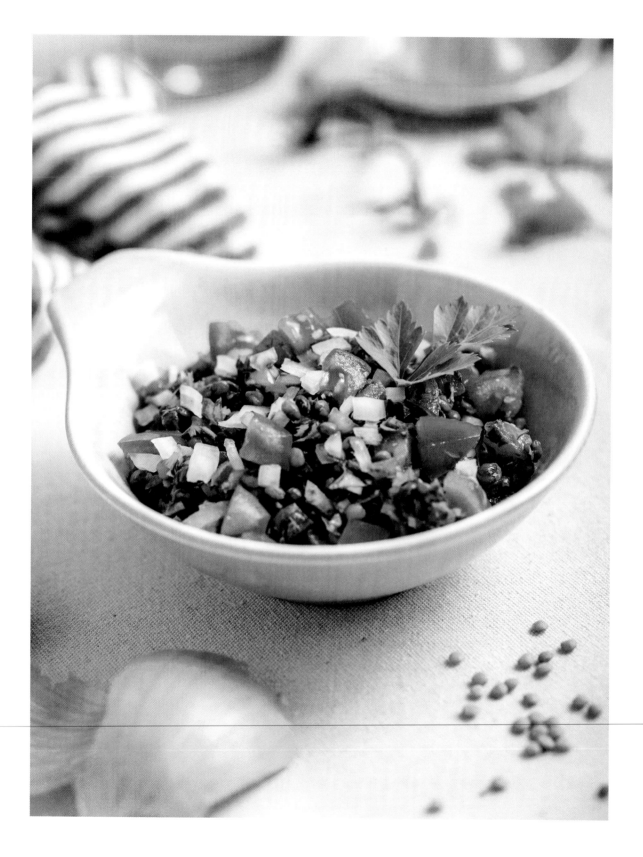

LENTIL TABBOULEH

PREP TIME: 20 min
COOK TIME: 0 min
TOTAL TIME: 20 min

MAKES 2 SERVINGS

This is our healthier version of the traditional Middle Eastern dish, tabbouleh. We simply replaced bulgur wheat with lentils (an incredibly powerful source of plant protein and one of my personal favorites) and transformed this into a protein-packed meal.

INGREDIENTS:

2 bunches curly parsley, minced (3 cups)

1 small onion, minced

2 tablespoons olive oil or to taste

2 limes, juiced

¼ teaspoon sea salt or to taste

2 15-ounce cans lentils, drained and rinsed (about 3 cups)

2 medium tomatoes, finely chopped

PREPARATION:

1. Thoroughly wash the parsley, shake off any excess water, and place the parsley on paper towels to dry.

2. Once the parsley is dry, discard the stems, and mound the parsley on a cutting board.

Tightly pack the parsley together, holding it down while slicing back and forth. Continue to tightly gather and chop until the parsley is fully minced.

3. In a mixing bowl, combine the onion, oil, lime juice, and sea salt and toss together.

4. Layer in the lentils, tomatoes, and freshly minced parsley.

5. Toss together until well combined, adjusting the taste if necessary, and serve.

TIP: This salad can be prepped in advance and stored for up to 2 days in the refrigerator. When ready to enjoy, simply toss together and serve!

PER SERVING: 553 calories, 31 grams protein, 81 grams carbohydrates, 16 grams total fat

BLACK BEAN BURRITO BOWL

PREP TIME: 25 min

COOK TIME: 30 min

TOTAL TIME: 55 min

MAKES 4 SERVINGS

This deconstructed burrito is a perfect plant-based meal. The Quinoa and black beans make a powerful protein combo while the peppers and Guacamole provide a great source of vitamins A, C, and E, fiber, folate, and heart-healthy fat.

INGREDIENTS:

2 cups cooked Quinoa (see recipe on page 343)

Pico de Gallo (see recipe on page 249) or 2 small tomatoes, lightly seeded and finely chopped

2 15-ounce cans black beans, drained and rinsed

1 large green bell pepper, washed, seeded, and finely chopped

Guacamole (see recipe on page 246)

Nacho Cheese (see recipe on page 339)

chives, for garnish

PREPARATION:

1. Prepare the Quinoa and Pico de Gallo.

2. Layer a serving bowl with the Quinoa, Pico de Gallo, black beans, peppers, and Guacamole.

3. Drizzle with Nacho Cheese, garnish with chives, and enjoy!

TIP: Leftovers can be stored in an airtight container for up to a few days.

PER SERVING: 329 calories, 17 grams protein, 58 grams carbohydrates, 5 grams total fat

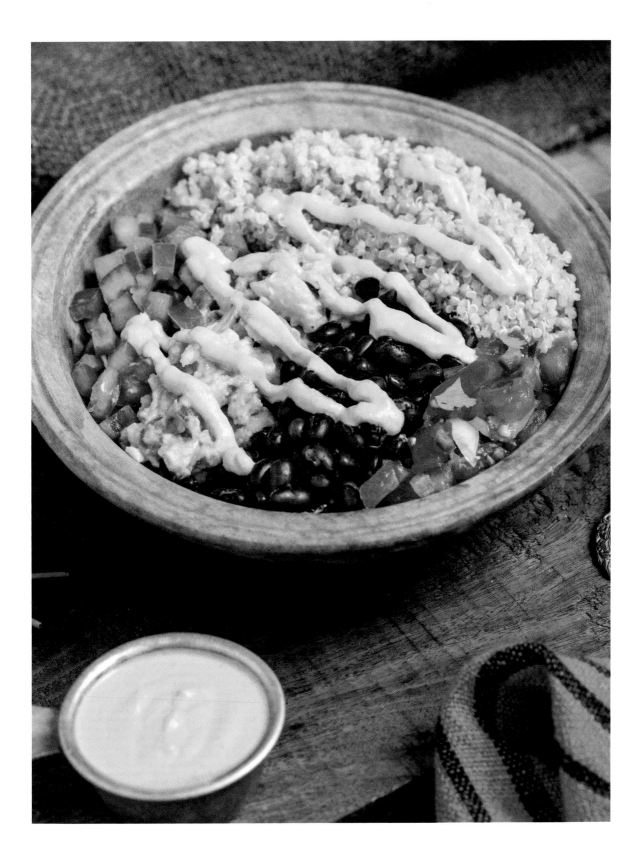

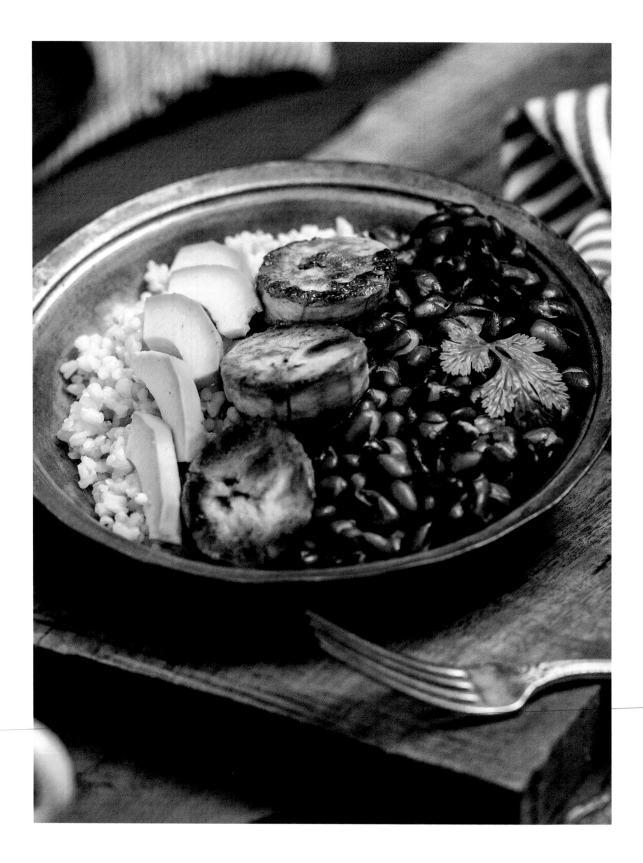

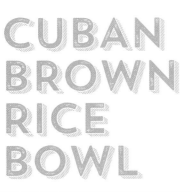

CUBAN BROWN RICE BOWL

PREP TIME: 15 min

COOK TIME: 55 min

TOTAL TIME: 70 min (does not include optional toppings)

MAKES 4 SERVINGS

This dish is a personal favorite because it brings back so many great memories of my childhood. (And what's not to love about black beans and rice?)

INGREDIENTS:

3 cups cooked Short-Grain Brown Rice (see recipe on page 319)

2 15-ounce cans black beans, rinsed and drained, or 3 cups cooked Black Beans (see recipe on page 315)

2 very ripe sweet plantains (Plátanos Maduros) (see recipe on page 253)

drizzle of Cashew Cheese (see recipe on page 320)

cilantro, for garnish

1 Hass avocado, halved, pitted, peeled, and sliced (optional)

Pico de Gallo (see recipe on page 249) (optional)

PREPARATION:

1. Prepare the Short-Grain Brown Rice, black beans, and Plátanos Maduros according to the recipes.

2. Assemble each bowl with ¾ cup of brown rice, about ¾ cup of black beans, plantains, and Cashew Cheese. Then garnish with cilantro and enjoy!

3. If you'd like, top the bowls with sliced avocados and/or Pico de Gallo.

PER SERVING: 464 calories, 17 grams protein, 95 grams carbohydrates, 4 grams total fat

MUSHROOM, SPINACH & QUINOA

PREP TIME: 20 min

COOK TIME: 35 min

TOTAL TIME: 55 min (does not include the Quinoa cook time)

MAKES 2 SERVINGS

According to wellness leader and expert Dr. Mercola, "mushrooms contain some of the most potent natural medicines on the planet. . . . Recent studies suggest anti-inflammatory characteristics that may be helpful for those suffering from asthma, rheumatoid arthritis, renal failure, and stroke damage."*

Mushrooms should be included more often in meals, because of their high nutritional value in vitamins, minerals and antioxidant phytonutrients. They're a good source of vitamin D_2, rich in B vitamins, concentrated in minerals like selenium and copper, and a good source of zinc and manganese.

The toasted pine nuts give this meal a nice crunch and balance all the flavors.

* http://articles.mercola.com/sites/articles/archive/2013/05/13/mushroom-benefits.aspx

INGREDIENTS:

2 tablespoons pine nuts

2 tablespoons canola oil or oil of choice

2 8-ounce mushroom packs, washed, and sliced

2 tablespoons coconut aminos

sea salt, to taste

1 15-ounce can chickpeas, rinsed and drained (about 1½ cups)

4 cups spinach

1 cup cooked Quinoa (see recipe on page 343)

PREPARATION:

1. Heat a dry skillet and cook the pine nuts over medium-low heat, stirring frequently, for about 3 minutes or until golden. Set aside.

2. Heat the oil in a saucepan or skillet over medium heat. Add the mushrooms, coconut aminos, and a pinch of salt and stir frequently for about 5 minutes until lightly browned. Make sure not to overcook the mushrooms to maximize their nutrients.

3. Add the chickpeas and spinach. Once the spinach begins to wilt, add the Quinoa and stir together for another few minutes. Taste and adjust the seasoning if necessary.

4. Serve and enjoy!

NOTE: Having a ready batch of premade Quinoa in the fridge each week comes in handy for recipes such as this one.

PER SERVING: 524 calories, 21 grams protein, 62 grams carbohydrates, 24 grams total fat

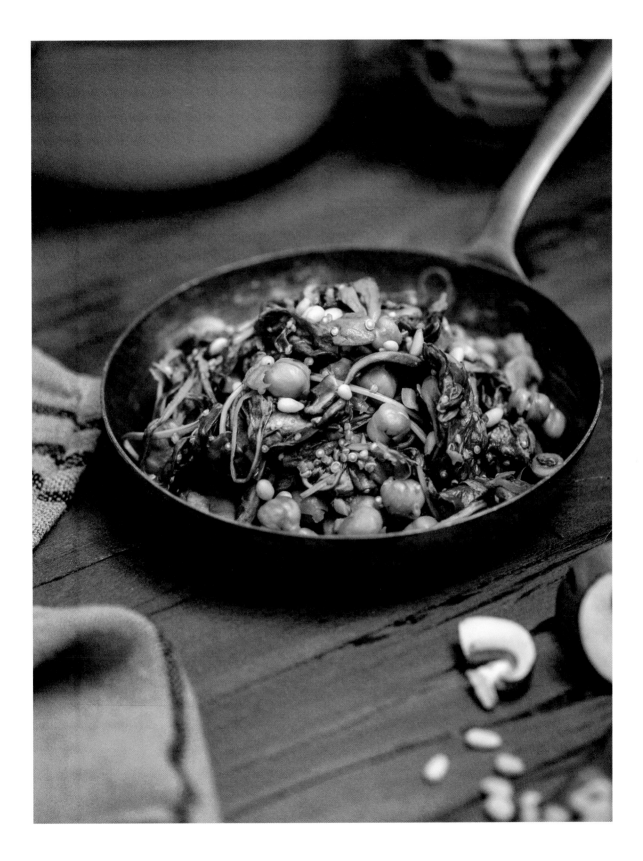

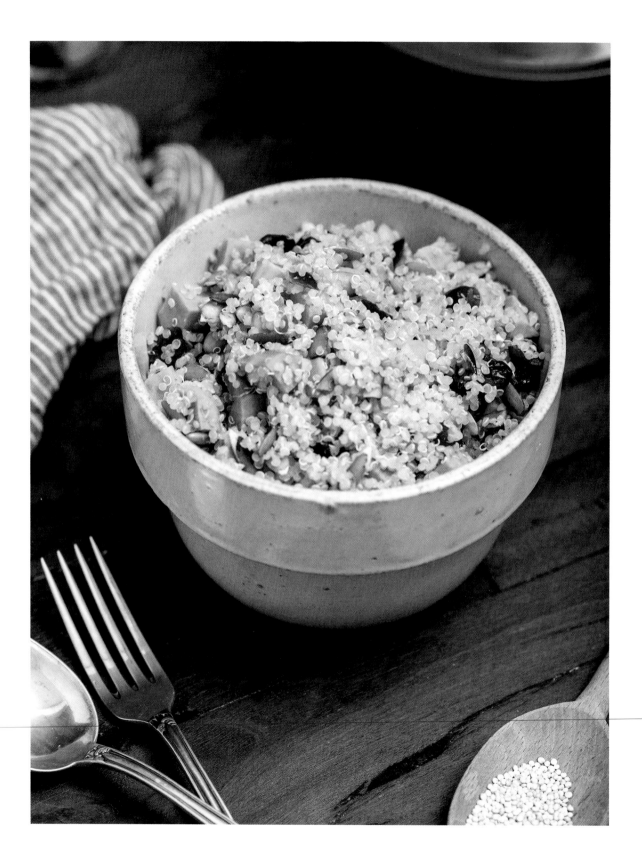

QUINOA & SWEET POTATO SALAD

PREP TIME: 10 min

COOK TIME: 15 min

TOTAL TIME: 25 min (does not include the Quinoa cook time)

MAKES 2 SERVINGS

The juxtaposition of flavors and textures makes this one of my all-time favorite salads. It's loaded with vitamins and minerals and rich in taste. Every ingredient used here has a uniquely powerful nutritional profile. Quinoa is one of a very few plant-based foods that is a complete protein source (contains all essential amino acids). Sweet potatoes are rich in vitamins A and C. Pumpkin seeds are loaded in zinc, magnesium, and heart-healthy omega-3 fatty acid. Cranberries are low in calories and known to reduce the risk of many cancers as well as urinary tract infections. With this much to offer in as little as four ingredients, this salad may very well become one of your all-time favorites.

INGREDIENTS:

1 small to medium-size sweet potato

1 cup cooked Quinoa (see recipe on page 343)

¼ cup pumpkin seeds (pepitas)

¼ cup dried cranberries

FOR THE DRESSING:

1 orange, juiced

1 lime, juiced

1 teaspoon Dijon mustard

fresh ground black pepper, to taste

pinch of sea salt, or to taste

PREPARATION:

1. Wash the sweet potato and cut it into cubes.

2. Steam for 15 minutes or until the sweet potatoes are fork tender throughout.

3. In a large bowl, toss the sweet potato, Quinoa, pumpkin seeds, and cranberries.

4. To prepare the dressing, whisk together the ingredients in a mixing bowl.

5. Drizzle the dressing over the quinoa bowl and toss together until well combined. Transfer to a serving bowl, season with fresh ground black pepper and enjoy.

PER SERVING: 403 calories, 11 grams protein, 70 grams carbohydrates, 10 grams total fat

QUINOA CRUNCH BOWL

PREP TIME: 30 min

COOK TIME: 30 min

TOTAL TIME: 60 min

MAKES 4 SERVINGS

Quinoa is a versatile and complete ingredient that's fun and easy to use in a multitude of recipes.

INGREDIENTS:

2 cups cooked Quinoa (see recipe on page 343)

2 large carrots, shredded (about 1½ cups)

1 15-ounce can black beans, drained and rinsed

1 small jicama, peeled and diced into ½-inch cubes (about 1 cup)

½ cup fresh parsley flakes

Lemon Dijon Vinaigrette Dressing (see recipe on page 335)

1 Hass avocado, halved, cored, peeled, and cut into cubes

2 tablespoons sunflower seeds, for garnish

PREPARATION:

1. Prepare the Quinoa and set aside to cool.

2. Peel or scrub the carrots, cut the ends off, then slice with a vegetable peeler or use a box grater to shred and transfer to a mixing bowl.

3. Add the Quinoa, black beans, jicama, parsley, and dressing to the mixing bowl and toss ingredients together.

4. Then add the diced avocados and gently toss again.

5. Serve, garnish with sunflower seeds, and enjoy!

PER SERVING: 398 calories, 13 grams protein, 54 grams carbohydrates, 17 grams total fat

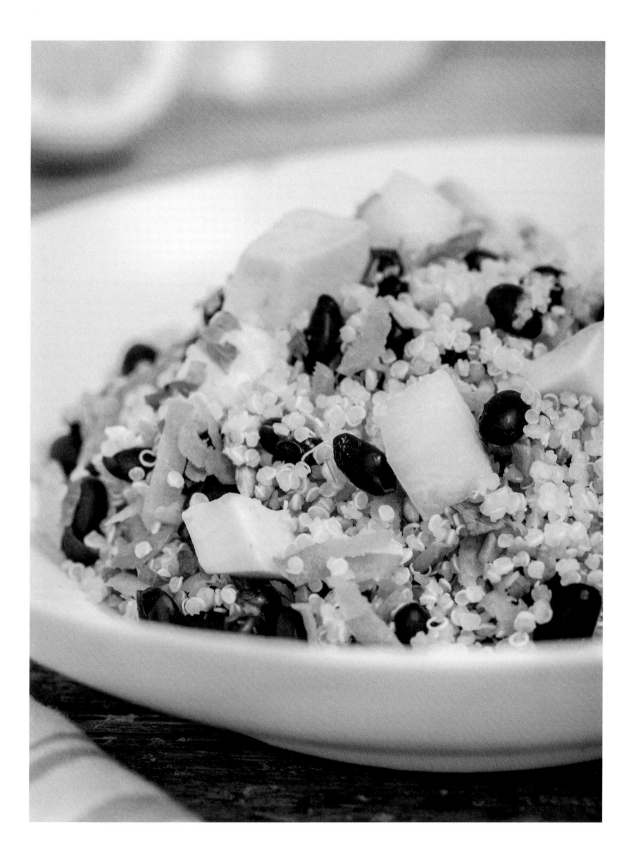

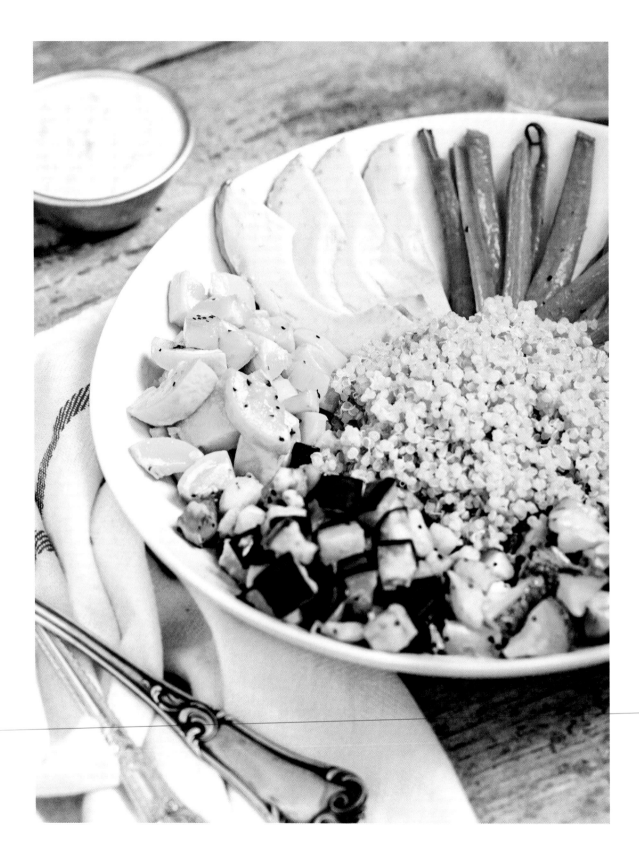

RAINBOW ROASTED VEGGIE BOWL

PREP TIME: 30 min

COOK TIME: 30 min

TOTAL TIME: 60 min

MAKES 4 SERVINGS

Here's a quick and easy way to enjoy all the benefits of a bowl of veggies without passing on flavor. The roasted sweet potato and carrots add a delicate touch of sweetness that is perfectly balanced by the avocado and quinoa. Perfect once topped with cashew cream.

INGREDIENTS:

2 cups cooked Quinoa (see recipe on page 343)

Cashew Cream Dressing (see recipe on page 323)

1 eggplant, washed and chopped

salt, to taste

1 large sweet potato, washed and chopped

1 large zucchini, washed, trimmed, and chopped

1 large summer squash, washed, trimmed, and chopped

2 large carrots, trimmed and sliced

1 tablespoon canola oil or oil of choice

sea salt, to taste

ground black pepper, to taste

1 Hass avocado, halved, cored, peeled, and sliced

PREPARATION:

1. Prepare the Quinoa and Cashew Cream Dressing and set aside.

2. Preheat oven to 400F and line a large baking sheet with parchment paper.

3. To prepare the eggplant, salt the pieces and arrange in a colander to remove the bitterness for about 15 minutes.

4. Rinse and dry with paper towels. Transfer the eggplant onto the baking sheet together with the sweet potato, zucchini, squash, and carrots. Lightly brush with oil, sea salt, and pepper and roast for about 25–30 minutes, tossing halfway through cooking time. Vegetables are ready when golden and tender. Make sure to watch closely to avoid burning.

5. Layer a serving bowl with the Quinoa, eggplant, sweet potato, zucchini, squash, and carrots, or simply toss all the ingredients together.

6. Then garnish with sliced avocado, drizzle with dressing, and enjoy immediately!

NOTE: For added protein, toss together with beans of your choice.

TIP: Leftovers can be stored in an airtight container for up to a few days.

PER SERVING: 414 calories, 13 grams protein, 51 grams carbohydrates, 20 grams total fat

VEGETABLE PAELLA

PREP TIME: 15 min

COOK TIME: 60 min

TOTAL TIME: 75 min (does not include Grandma's Go-To Tomato Sauce cook time)

MAKES 4 SERVINGS

Paella is a traditional Spanish rice dish known as a mixture of rice, beans, seafood, and meat. We've kept the tradition alive with this vegetable variation. It's rich in flavor, and the textures and nutritional value make it a family favorite.

INGREDIENTS:

1 cup Grandma's Go-To Tomato Sauce (see recipe on page 331)

1 tablespoon canola oil

1 teaspoon garlic, minced

½ onion, minced

1 small red pepper, washed, cored, seeded, and finely chopped

¾ cup frozen peas

1 15-ounce can chickpeas, drained and rinsed (about 1½ cups)

1¼ cups uncooked short-grain brown rice

3 cups vegetable broth, unsalted, add more if necessary

2 teaspoons smoked paprika

1 teaspoon ground turmeric

1 teaspoon ground cumin

1 teaspoon sea salt or to taste

ground black pepper, to taste

1 lime, quartered, for garnish

fresh parsley, for garnish

PREPARATION:

1. Prepare Grandma's Go-to Tomato Sauce and set aside while preparing remaining ingredients.

2. Heat oil in a large skillet over medium heat and sauté the garlic, onions, and peppers until golden.

3. Add the tomato sauce, frozen peas, and chickpeas and cook for another few minutes.

4. Add the rice, vegetable broth, smoked paprika, turmeric, cumin, sea salt, and pepper.

5. Stir together until well combined and bring to a boil.

6. Bring down the heat to medium low, cover, and let the mixture cook for about 45 minutes. If the liquid has evaporated, but the rice is still dry, add more vegetable broth and cook for another 10 minutes.

7. Once the rice is cooked, remove it from the heat and let it sit for another few minutes, covered.

8. Garnish with lime wedges and parsley and serve.

TIP: Leftovers can be stored in an airtight container in the refrigerator up to a week.

PER SERVING: 430 calories, 12 grams protein, 80 grams carbohydrates, 7 grams total fat

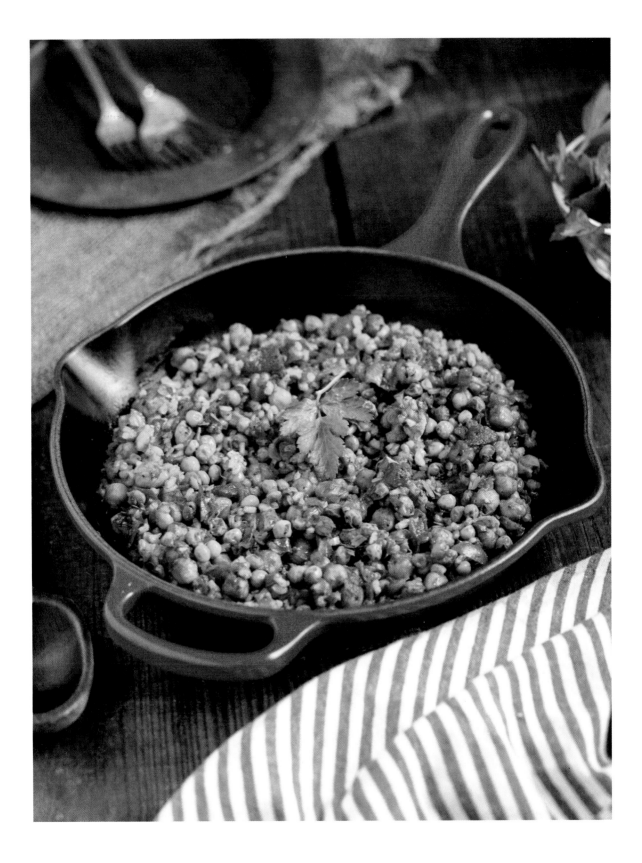

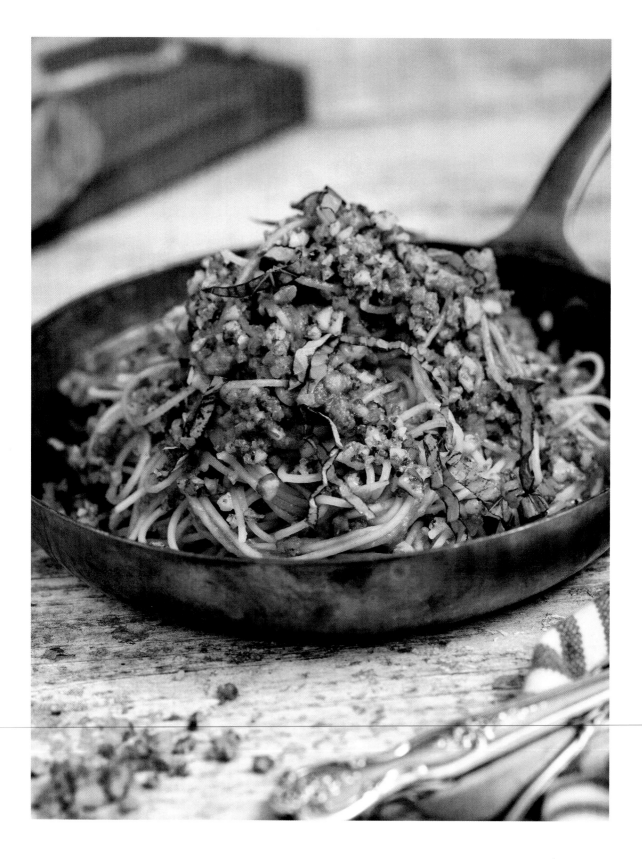

BOLOGNESE PASTA

PREP TIME: 20 min

COOK TIME: 35 min

TOTAL TIME: 55 min

MAKES 4 SERVINGS

This one is an amalgamation of some of my favorites (walnut meat, tomato sauce, parmesan) that makes another favorite. It can also be made using raw spiralized veggie pasta for a lighter dish.

INGREDIENTS:

1 8-ounce package uncooked gluten-free angel hair pasta or linguine

4 cups Grandma's Go-To Tomato Sauce (see recipe on page 331)

1 cup Walnut Meat (see recipe on page 347)

Parmesan Cheese, to taste (see recipe on page 340)

PREPARATION:

1. Bring a large pot of salted water to a boil, and cook the pasta according to package directions.

2. In a saucepan, combine the Grandma's Go-To Tomato Sauce and Walnut Meat and cook over medium-low heat for about 5–10 minutes.

3. Transfer the pasta to the saucepan and toss together to combine. Serve with a sprinkling of Parmesan Cheese and enjoy!

PER SERVING: 363 calories, 9 grams protein, 59 grams carbohydrates, 12 grams total fat

EGGPLANT ROLLATINI

PREP TIME: 30 min

COOK TIME: 45 min

TOTAL TIME: 75 min

MAKES 2 SERVINGS

I've always loved Italian food, and rollatini is no exception. But after I gave up dairy years ago, I almost gave up this dish as well. This recipe changed everything.

INGREDIENTS:

salt, to taste

1 large eggplant, washed and thinly sliced lengthwise (8–10 slices)

4 cups raw spinach

sea salt, to taste

2 cups Grandma's Go-To Tomato Sauce (see recipe on page 331)

1 tomato, washed and thinly sliced

8 tablespoons Cashew Cheese (see recipe on page 320)

1 cup shredded carrot

5 cherry tomatoes, washed and halved

dried basil leaves, to taste

dried oregano leaves, to taste

ground black pepper, to taste

PREPARATION:

1. Salt the eggplant slices and arrange in a colander to remove the bitterness for about 15 minutes.

2. Preheat oven to 375F.

3. Rinse the eggplant slices well and dry with paper towels. Place the slices on a baking sheet and bake for about 20 minutes.

4. In a lightly greased skillet, over medium-high heat, sauté the spinach for about 5 minutes with a pinch of sea salt until completely wilted. Set aside.

5. In a baking dish (8" x 8"), add about 1 cup of tomato sauce, then layer with the sliced tomato and set aside.

6. Scoop about 2 teaspoons to 1 tablespoon of the spinach, Cashew Cheese, and carrot onto each eggplant slice and roll it up, placing the end facing down on the baking dish. Continue rolling until all eggplant slices are used. Top with more tomato sauce, cherry tomatoes, basil, oregano, sea salt, and pepper.

7. Bake for about 20 minutes until eggplant is slightly browned.

8. Serve and enjoy!

PER SERVING: 333 calories, 14 grams protein, 47 grams carbohydrates, 14 grams total fat

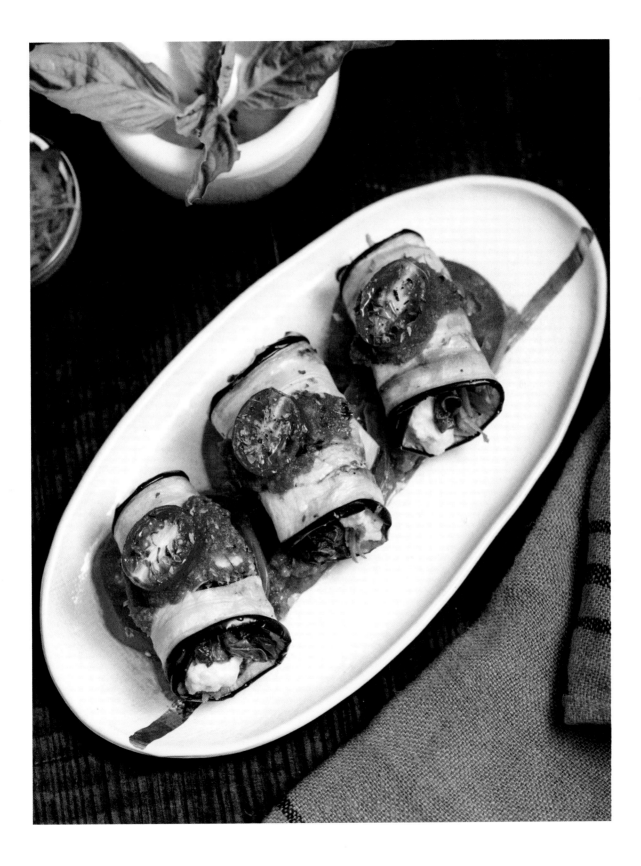

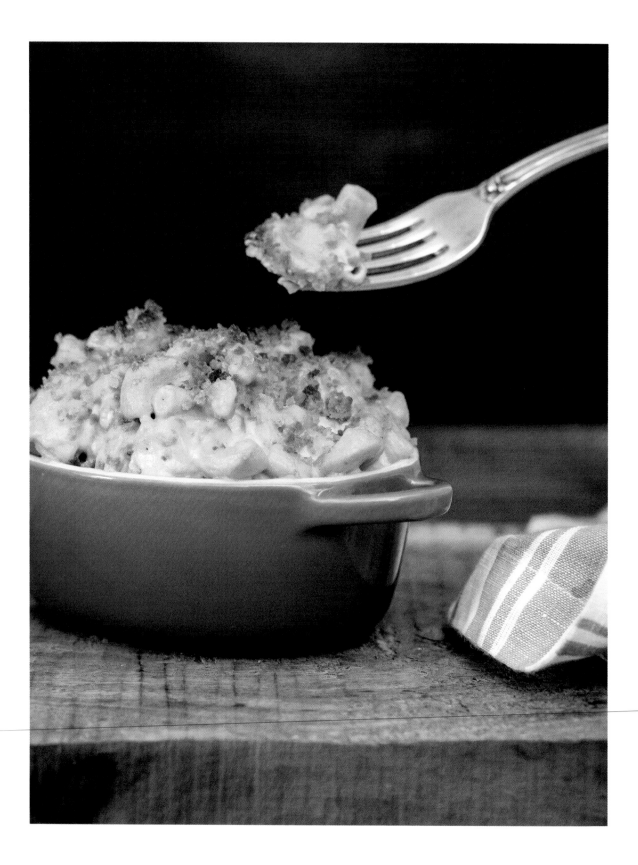

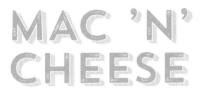

MAC 'N' CHEESE

PREP TIME: 10 min

COOK TIME: 10 min

TOTAL TIME: 20 min

MAKES 4 SERVINGS

This incredibly simple dish will satisfy even the pickiest kids and also makes a mean, guilt-free weekend indulgence.

INGREDIENTS:

Cashew Cheese (see recipe on page 320)

2 teaspoons ground turmeric

sea salt, to taste

10 ounces uncooked gluten-free elbow pasta

scallions, for garnish (optional)

PREPARATION:

1. Prepare the Cashew Cheese according to the recipe and mix with 2 teaspoons of turmeric. Set aside while preparing the pasta.

2. Bring a large pot of salted water to a boil.

3. Add the pasta and cook according to the package instructions.

4. Drain the pasta, reserving one cup of the pasta water, and return the cooked pasta to the pot.

5. Gently stir in the cheese sauce, adding the pasta water as needed until the sauce is as thick or thin as you'd like.

6. Spoon Mac 'n' Cheese into bowls and enjoy!

PER SERVING: 502 calories, 14 grams protein, 69 grams carbohydrates, 21 grams total fat

PENNE PASTA WITH SPINACH CREAM SAUCE

PREP TIME: 10 min
COOK TIME: 10 min
TOTAL TIME: 20 min

MAKES 4 SERVINGS

People often ask me if plant-based diets recommend avoiding pasta. My answer is almost always the same. It's not pasta as a dish that is the problem but rather the ingredients used in preparing it. Choose dairy-free and gluten-free pasta that is minimally processed for taste that doesn't lack in nutrition and prepare it with fresh veggies (organic, whenever possible) and homemade sauces for optimum flavor and nutrient density.

INGREDIENTS:

pinch of sea salt

10 ounces uncooked gluten-free penne pasta

1 5-ounce package baby spinach

Cashew Cream Sauce (see recipe on page 323)

2 tablespoons pine nuts or to taste

PREPARATION:

1. Bring a large pot of salted water to a boil. Add the pasta and cook according to package directions.

2. In a food processor, process the spinach. Then add the Cashew Cream Sauce and pulse together until well combined.

3. Drain the pasta, reserving 1 cup of the cooking water, and return the cooked pasta to the pot.

4. Add the sauce to the pot and gently toss together with the pasta.

5. Taste and adjust seasoning, if necessary. To thin the sauce, add water ¼ of a cup at a time until the sauce has reached desired consistency.

6. Serve and garnish with pine nuts!

PER SERVING: 409 calories, 11 grams protein, 63 grams carbohydrates, 14 grams total fat

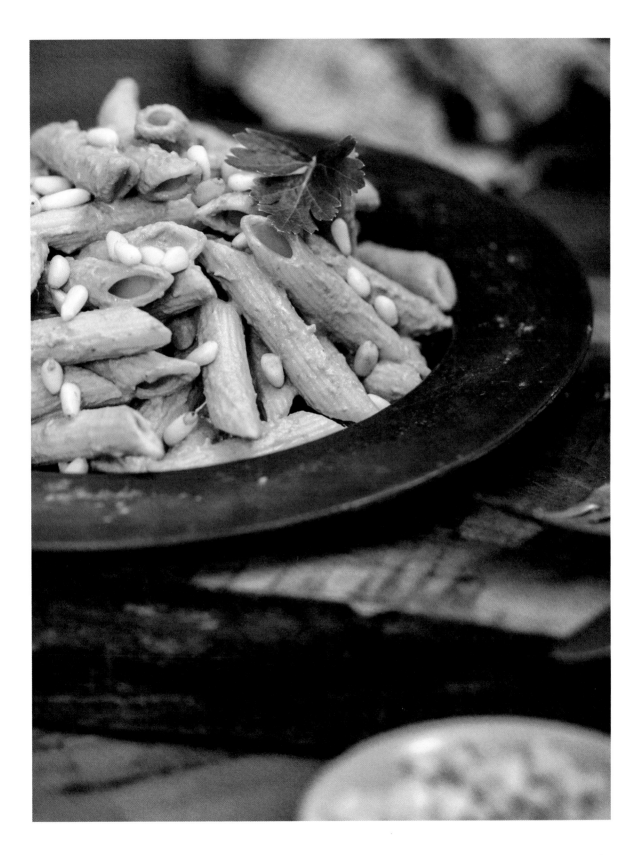

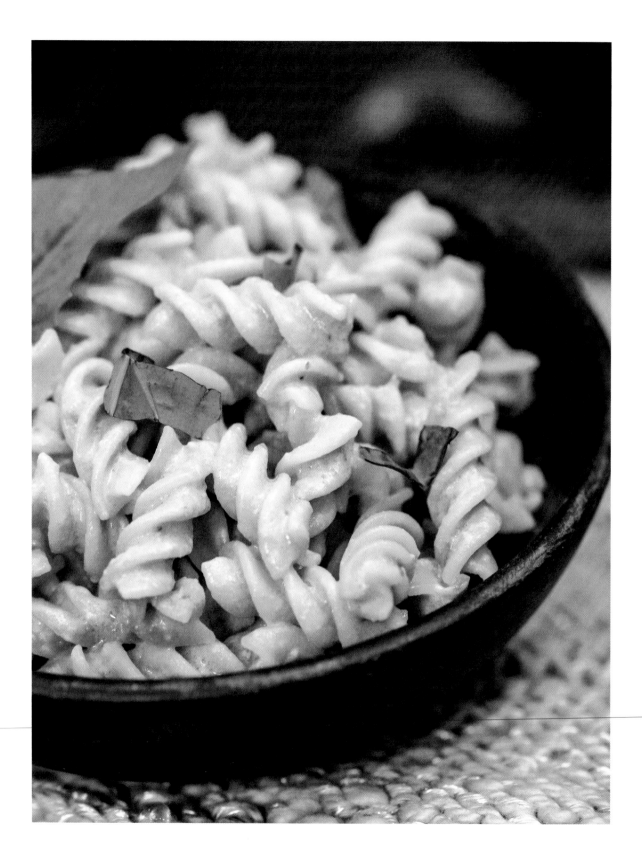

TOMATO BASIL CREAM PASTA

PREP TIME: 20 min

COOK TIME: 10 min

TOTAL TIME: 30 min

MAKES 4 SERVINGS

This is a dish that delights even the harshest critics, without the common allergens gluten and dairy, which often irritate the digestive system. Go ahead and enjoy your pasta again.

INGREDIENTS:

¼–½ teaspoon sea salt or to taste

10 ounces uncooked gluten-free pasta, fusilli, or other spiral pasta

1 teaspoon olive oil

¼ small onion, diced

2 large tomatoes, cored and chopped

4 basil leaves, roughly chopped, with some set aside for garnish

¼ cup water, to thin sauce (optional)

1 cup Cashew Cream Sauce (see recipe on page 323)

Parmesan Cheese, to taste (see recipe on page 340)

PREPARATION:

1. Bring a large pot of salted water to a boil.

2. Add the pasta and cook according to the package directions.

3. Add the olive oil to a saucepan, over medium-high heat, and sauté the onion for a few minutes with a dash of salt until the onion is translucent.

4. In a food processor or blender, process the tomato, basil, Cashew Cream Sauce, onion, and ¼ teaspoon salt until the sauce reaches a creamy consistency. Then pour the sauce from the blender to the saucepan, stir, and let cook for about 5 minutes at a simmer. To thin the sauce, add a few tablespoons of water at a time, until desired consistency is reached.

5. Rinse and drain the pasta and return the pasta to the pot.

6. Pour the sauce into the pot and gently toss together with the pasta. Taste and adjust seasoning, if necessary.

7. Serve with a sprinkling of Parmesan Cheese and basil!

PER SERVING: 466 calories, 13 grams protein, 69 grams carbohydrates, 17 grams total fat

REBOOT PLATE

PREP TIME: 20 min

COOK TIME: 30 min

TOTAL TIME: 50 min

MAKES 2 SERVINGS

This dish is amazingly powerful and loaded with phytochemicals for an instant reboot that will reset your digestive system and recharge your body. I love the reboot plate at least once a week and sometimes even opt for it a couple of days in a row.

INGREDIENTS:

1 cup cooked Quinoa (see recipe on page 343)

2 cups small broccoli florets

1 cup carrots, roughly chopped

½ cup celery, diced

2 tablespoons almonds, sliced

2 tablespoons sunflower seeds

2 tablespoons pumpkin seeds (pepitas)

1 lemon, juiced

sea salt, to taste

ground black pepper, to taste

1 Hass avocado, halved, pitted, peeled, and sliced

microgreens, for garnish

PREPARATION:

1. Add cooked quinoa to a mixing bowl and set aside.

2. In a food processor, pulse the broccoli until it reaches a crumbly consistency. Scoop the broccoli crumbs into the mixing bowl.

3. Pulse the carrots until crumbly and add them to the broccoli-quinoa bowl. Toss in the celery, almonds, sunflower seeds, and pumpkins seeds.

4. Sprinkle in the lemon juice, sea salt, and pepper and toss the ingredients until well combined.

5. Gently fold in the avocado, garnish with microgreens, and serve.

PER SERVING: 407 calories, 14 grams protein, 41 grams carbohydrates, 24 grams total fat

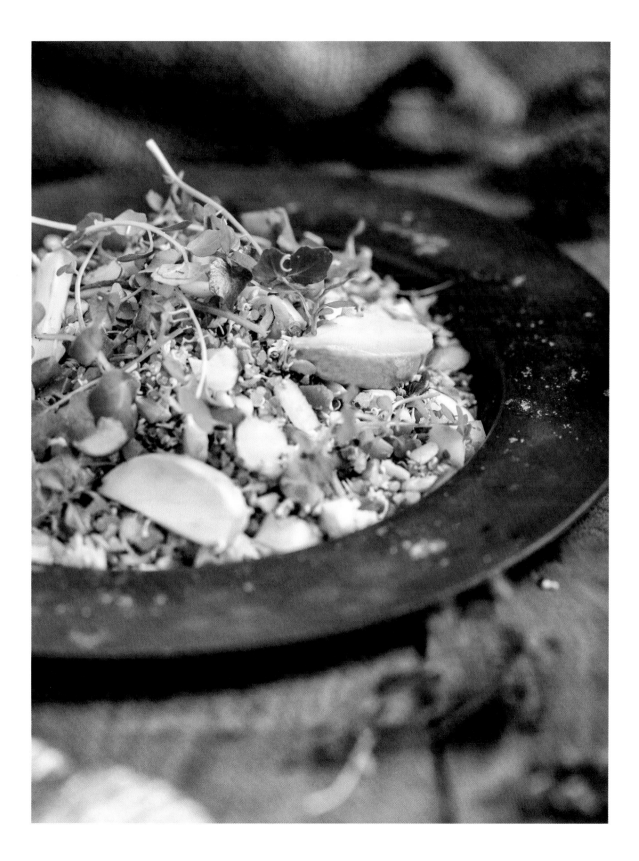

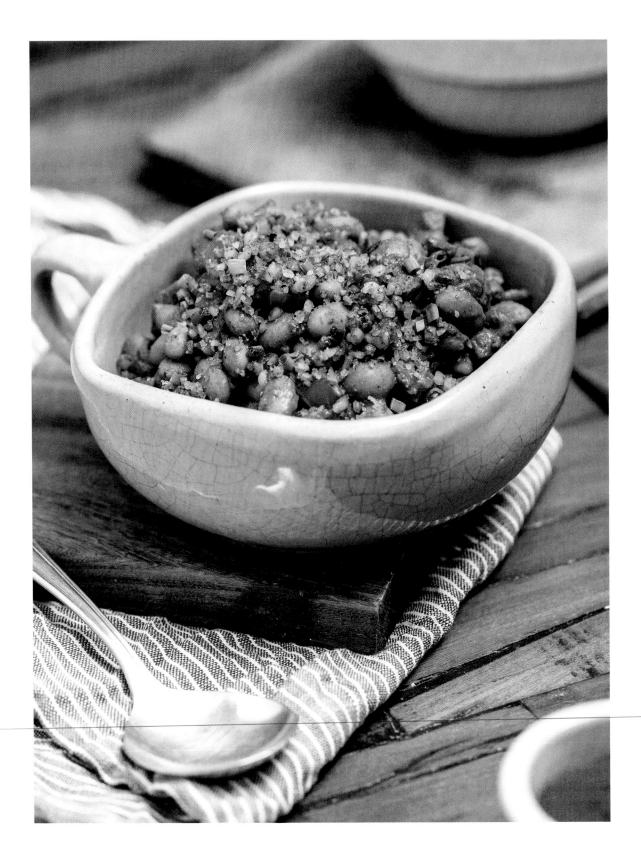

WALNUT CHILI

PREP TIME: 20 min

COOK TIME: 90 min

TOTAL TIME: 110 min

MAKES 4 SERVINGS

This delicious protein-packed chili is a smash in our home!

INGREDIENTS:

1 cup pinto beans, presoaked overnight in 3–4 cups water

1½ cups water

½ cup Walnut Meat, for garnish (see recipe on page 347)

1 tablespoon canola oil

¼ cup white onion, finely chopped

¾ teaspoon sea salt or to taste

1 large red bell pepper, halved, seeded, and diced (about 1 cup)

1 large tomato, washed and diced (about 1 cup)

2 tablespoons parsley flakes

1 tablespoon ground cumin

1 teaspoon paprika

1 teaspoon chili powder

½ teaspoon dried oregano

½ teaspoon turmeric powder

¼ teaspoon garlic powder

cayenne pepper, to taste (optional)

diced chives, or fresh cilantro, for garnish

PREPARATION:

1. Rinse and drain the beans.

2. Add the beans to a pot and add enough water to cover them by ½ inch, and bring to a boil.

3. Reduce to medium-low heat, cover and let simmer for 60–90 minutes. If necessary, add more water.

4. Meanwhile, prepare the Walnut Meat and set it aside. When the beans are just about tender, heat the oil in a skillet over medium-high and sauté the onions with a pinch of salt for 5 minutes until translucent.

5. Stir in the peppers and tomatoes together with remaining ingredients (except for the Walnut Meat and chives). Cover the mixture and cook for another 5 minutes.

6. Adjust the spices, if necessary.

7. When the desired tenderness is reached, serve the chili and garnish it with the Walnut Meat and chives, and enjoy!

OPTION:

▶ Try adding diced avocados and/or Cashew Cheese (see recipe on page 320) for a creamier flavor or enjoy with sriracha sauce for extra heat!

PER SERVING: 319 calories, 14 grams protein, 39 grams carbohydrates, 13 grams total fat

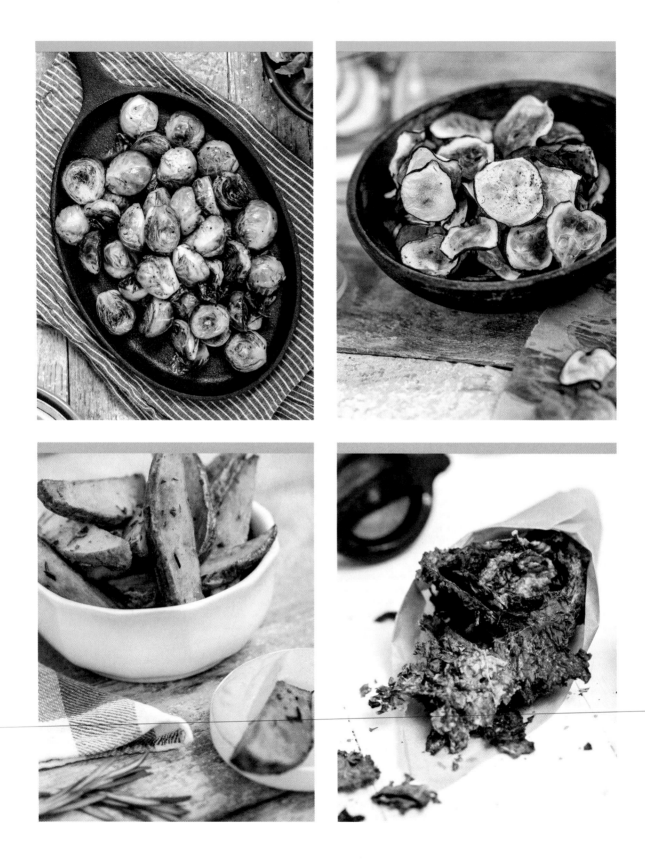

SNACKS AND SIDES

SOMETIMES YOU JUST NEED a little pick-me-up in the middle of a busy afternoon or before a workout to raise those energy levels.

As an afternoon snack or to serve to your friends and family at your next party, these dips and sides are versatile, delicious, and, of course, healthy. Dips and sides are often complete meals, pairing perfectly with our Light or Indulgent Entrées. These recipes are our favorites and are sure to delight your family and guests.

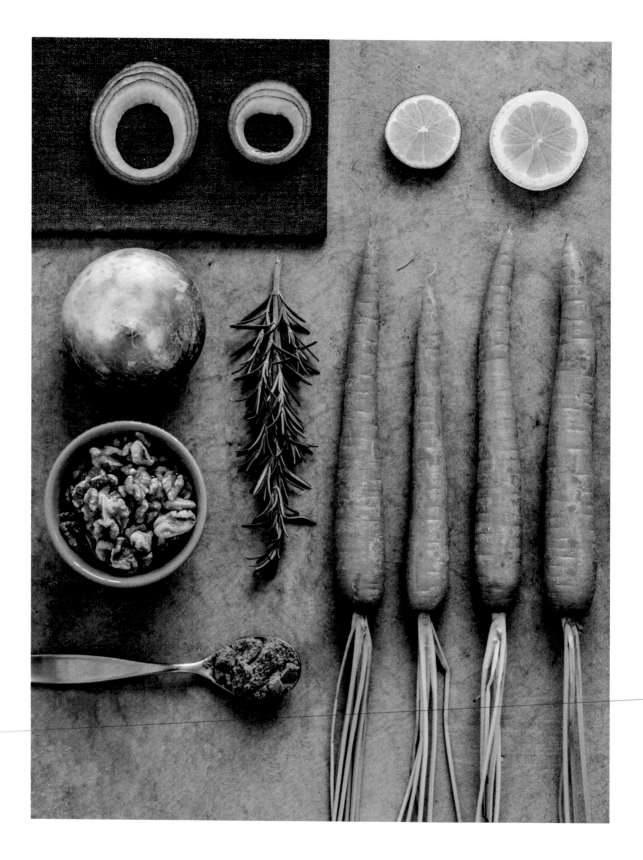

LIGHT SNACKS AND SIDES

(UNDER 150 CALORIES)

LIGHT

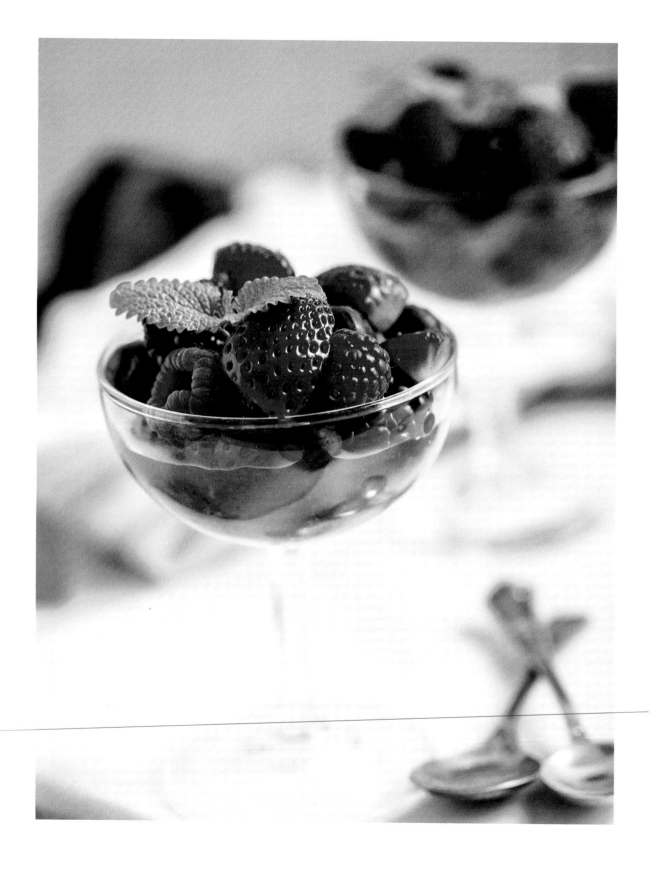

BERRY COCKTAIL

PREP TIME: 10 min
COOK TIME: 0 min
TOTAL TIME: 10 min

MAKES 4 SERVINGS

This could very easily be called an antioxidant cocktail because it's loaded with antioxidants for optimum health while still tasting and looking very much like a delicious dessert.

INGREDIENTS:

1 cup fresh strawberries, washed, hulled, and quartered lengthwise

1 cup fresh blueberries, washed

1 cup fresh blackberries, washed

1 cup raspberries, washed

3–4 fresh oranges, squeezed (about 1 cup)

fresh mint, for garnish

PREPARATION:

1. Evenly divide the berries into 4 serving glasses.

2. Pour freshly squeezed orange juice into each glass, garnish with mint, and enjoy!

TIP: You can also top this recipe with a scoop of Coconut Whipped Cream (see recipe on page 324). Leftovers can be stored in an airtight container for up to a few days.

PER SERVING: 92 calories, 2 grams protein, 22 grams carbohydrates, 1 gram total fat

LIGHT

FROZEN BANANA & SUNFLOWER BUTTER PIE

PREP TIME: 5 min

COOK TIME: 0 min

TOTAL TIME: 2 hrs 5 min

MAKES 2 SERVINGS

Here's a two-ingredient treat that's super simple—and a kid favorite!

INGREDIENTS:

1 ripe banana

1 tablespoon sunflower butter

PREPARATION:

1. Peel the banana, place it in a small bowl, and mash with a fork.

2. Place the mashed banana into a molded freezer tray (or simply shape it into the desired form by hand). Place the shaped bananas on parchment paper and store until frozen.

3. Remove the shaped bananas from the freezer and spread them with sunflower butter. Freeze again.

4. Allow the treats to harden before removing from the freezer to serve.

PER SERVING: 102 calories, 2 grams protein, 15 grams carbohydrates, 5 grams total fat

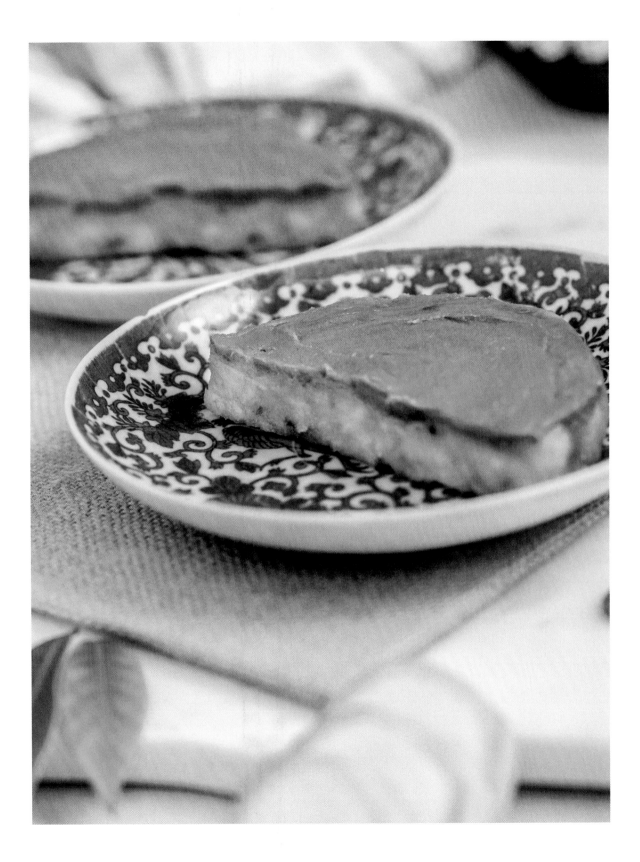

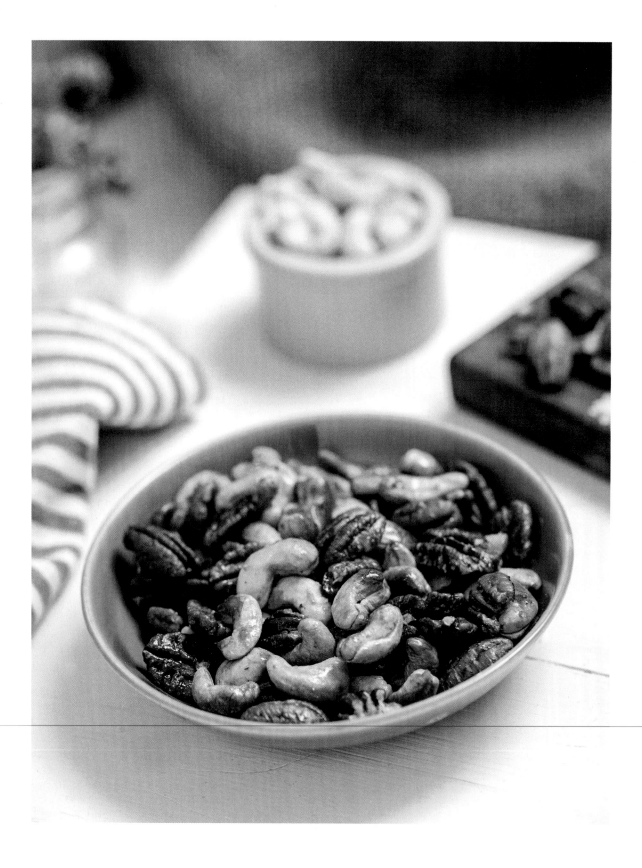

CANDIED PECANS & CASHEWS

PREP TIME: 5 min

COOK TIME: 10 min

TOTAL TIME: 15 min

MAKES 8 SERVINGS

It's a good thing this recipe is quick and easy to make because once your family has tasted it, you'll soon find an empty container wherever it was stored.

INGREDIENTS:

¼ cup pecans

¼ cup cashews

1 tablespoon maple syrup

pinch of sea salt

pinch of fresh ground pepper

PREPARATION:

1. Preheat oven to 350F.

2. Place all the ingredients in an ovenproof bowl and toss until the nuts are evenly coated.

3. Place mix into the oven for 7–8 minutes or until the syrup has dried up.

4. Remove the nuts from the oven. Once cool, carefully break up the nuts and enjoy!

NOTE: This recipe can also be made with just one preferred nut of choice by substituting pecans for the ¼ cup of cashews or vice versa.

PER SERVING: 57 calories, 1 gram protein, 4 grams carbohydrates, 5 grams total fat

LIGHT

CRISP BREAD CRACKERS

PREP TIME: 10 min

COOK TIME: 45 min

TOTAL TIME: 55 min

MAKES 8 CRACKERS

Enjoy this crispy cracker as a snack by topping it with your favorite plant-based options!

INGREDIENTS:

¼ cup almond meal/flour

½ cup gluten-free oat flour

1½ tablespoons pumpkin seeds, divided

1½ tablespoons sunflower seeds, divided

2 tablespoons flax meal

½ cup water

¼ teaspoon sea salt or to taste

PREPARATION:

1. Preheat oven to 325F. Line a baking sheet with parchment paper.

2. In a bowl, combine and mix all the ingredients (except for 1 tablespoon pumpkin seeds, 1 tablespoon sunflower seeds, and the salt).

3. Let mixture sit for 5–10 minutes so that the liquid is absorbed and the dough thickens.

4. Thinly spread the dough onto the baking sheet with the back of a spoon and sprinkle with the remaining pumpkin seeds, sunflower seeds, and salt.

5. Carefully cut the dough into 8 rectangles, using a knife. Feel free to cut the dough into smaller portions.

6. Bake for about 45 minutes or until the crackers are golden brown and crisp.

7. Let cool and enjoy!

TIP: Completely cooled leftovers can be stored in an airtight container at room temperature for up to a week. The cracker dough can also be premade and wrapped in plastic wrap in the refrigerator for up to a few days. When ready to enjoy, simply follow the preparation steps.

PER SERVING: 73 calories, 3 grams protein, 7 grams carbohydrates, 4 grams total fat

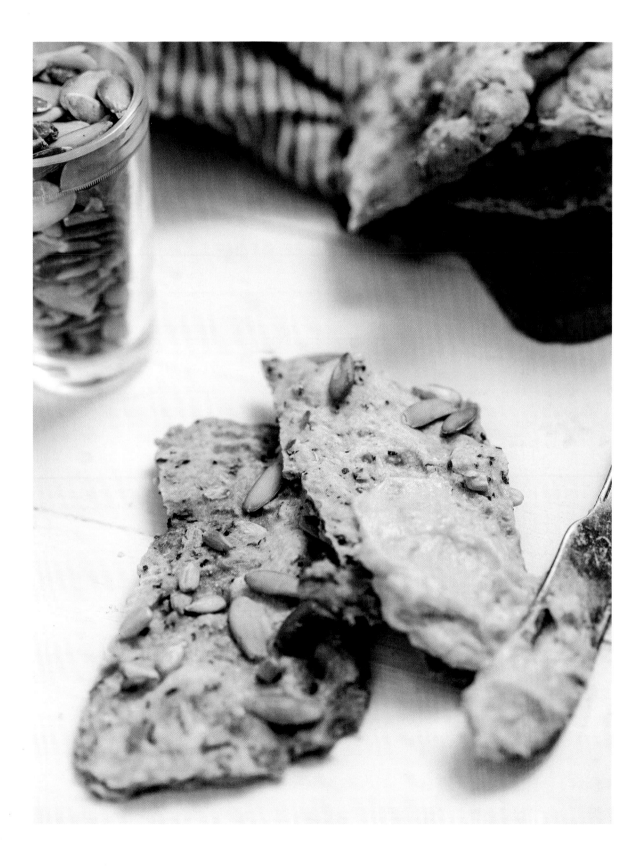

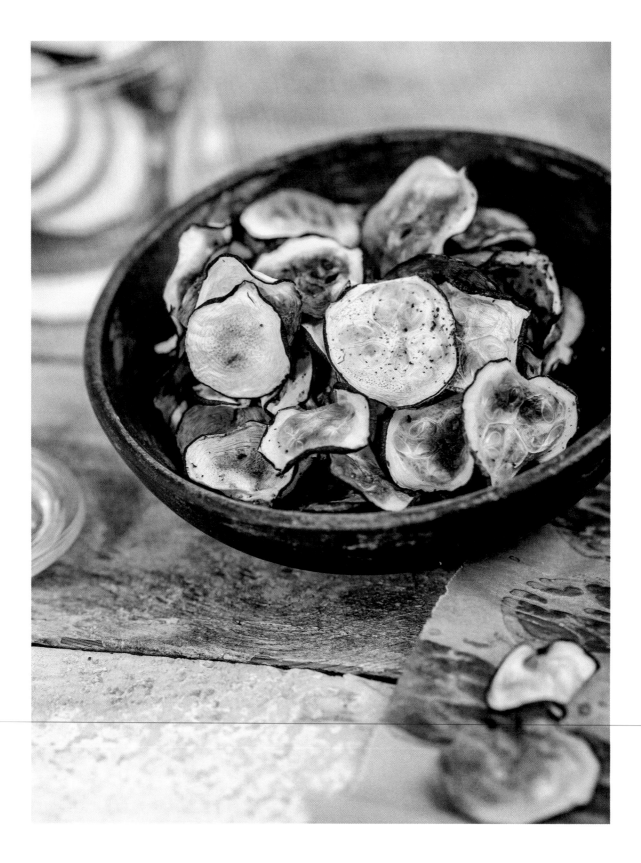

SALT & VINEGAR ZUCCHINI CHIPS

PREP TIME: 5 min

COOK TIME: 20 min

TOTAL TIME: 25 min (or up to 12 hours if prepared in a dehydrator)

MAKES 1 SERVING

Zucchini chips are a healthy alternative to commercial chips. We love preparing these using our dehydrator, but they can easily be made in an oven.

INGREDIENTS:

1 large zucchini

white vinegar, for soaking

dash of sea salt

freshly ground black pepper, to taste

PREPARATION:

1. Preheat oven to 350F.

2. Line a large baking dish with parchment paper.

3. Slice the zucchini into ⅛-inch-thick rounds.

4. In a mixing bowl, submerge the zucchini slices in white vinegar and let them soak for 30 minutes.

5. Pour the vinegar from the bowl and drain the zucchini well. Toss the zucchini slices with sea salt and freshly ground pepper.

6. Bake the zucchini until crisp, approximately 20 minutes. (Monitor the zucchini, because every oven is different.) Enjoy.

NOTE: These chips can also be made in a dehydrator, but would take considerably longer to prepare.

PER SERVING: 58 calories, 4 grams protein, 10 grams carbohydrates, 1 gram total fat

CRUNCHY CHICKPEAS

PREP TIME: 10 min

COOK TIME: 35 min

TOTAL TIME: 45 min

MAKES 4 SERVINGS

I've always loved chickpeas, and there's something about a good crunch that is very satisfying. Here, we have the best of both worlds in a guilt-free snack!

INGREDIENTS:

1 15-ounce can chickpeas, rinsed and drained

1 tablespoon extra-virgin olive oil

½ teaspoon garlic powder

½ teaspoon sea salt or to taste

ground black pepper, to taste

PREPARATION:

1. Preheat oven to 400F. Line a baking sheet with parchment paper.

2. Rinse and drain the chickpeas in a colander, discarding the thin skin of the beans. Pat dry the chickpeas thoroughly, removing as much moisture as possible. This helps to achieve a crispier texture.

3. In a medium bowl, toss the chickpeas with the oil, garlic powder, sea salt, and pepper.

4. Scatter the seasoned chickpeas on baking sheet and bake for about 35 minutes until crisp and golden, tossing them occasionally to make sure they don't burn. Chickpeas will continue to get crunchy as they cool.

5. Let the chickpeas cool completely and set them aside until ready to enjoy or store in an airtight container at room temperature. They are best when eaten within a day or two.

PER SERVING: 110 calories, 4 grams protein, 13 grams carbohydrates, 5 grams total fat

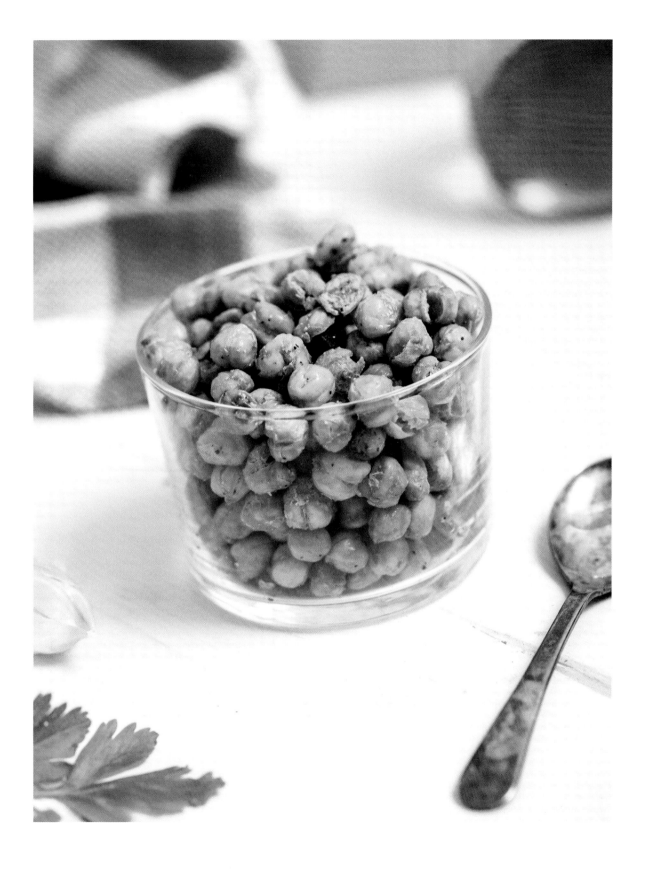

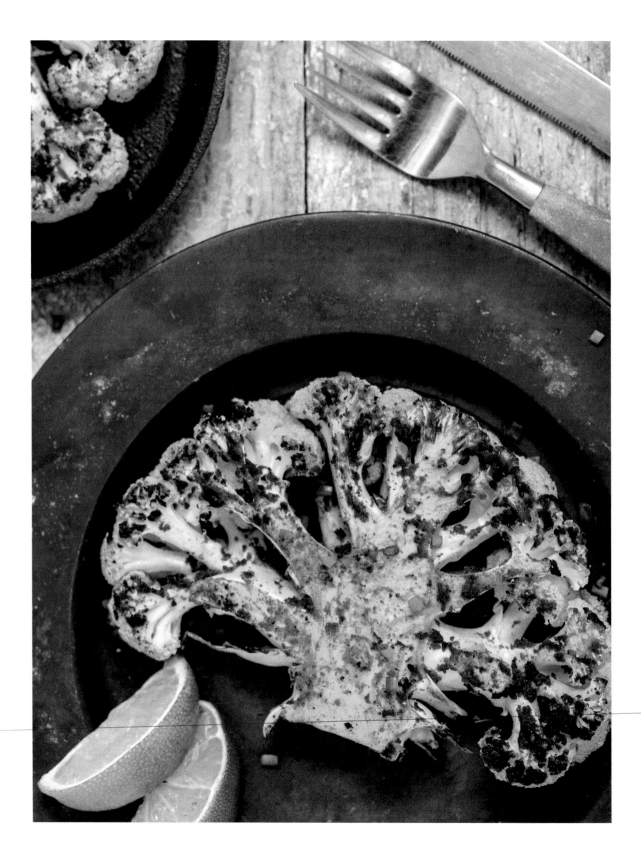

CURRY CAULIFLOWER STEAK

PREP TIME: 5 min
COOK TIME: 20 min
TOTAL TIME: 25 min

MAKES 4 SERVINGS

Cauliflower is an immune-boosting vegetable packed with antioxidants, fiber, and vitamins C and K, which may help reduce inflammation.

INGREDIENTS:

1 large head cauliflower

2 tablespoons coconut oil, melted

1 tablespoon curry powder

1 tablespoon ground paprika

1 teaspoon ground cumin

1 teaspoon ground turmeric

½ lime, juiced

¼–½ teaspoon sea salt or to taste

chives, for garnish

scallions, for garnish

lime wedges, to serve

DIRECTIONS:

1. Preheat oven to 450F and line a baking sheet with parchment paper.

2. Wash and cut the cauliflower from top center, slicing into at least 4 1-inch-thick slices. Save the florets that fall apart to prepare another recipe like Cheesy Cauliflower (see page 270) or simply roast together with the steaks.

3. In a bowl, combine the oil, spices, lime juice, and salt and evenly brush on both sides of the cauliflower steaks.

4. Place the steaks on the baking sheet and bake for 15–20 minutes until golden.

5. Serve, garnished with chives, scallions, lime wedges, and enjoy!

PER SERVING: 129 calories, 5 grams protein, 14 grams carbohydrates, 8 grams total fat

GUACAMOLE

PREP TIME: 10 min

COOK TIME: 0 min

TOTAL TIME: 10 min

MAKES 2 SERVINGS

Enjoy this guacamole simply as a dip with chips or as a side dish with many of our recipes, like the Black Bean, Sweet Potato & Quinoa Salad (see recipe on page 167).

INGREDIENTS:

1 Hass avocado, pitted, peeled, and chopped

½ lime, juiced, or more to taste

¼ teaspoon sea salt, to taste

2 tablespoons tomato, seeded and finely diced

2 tablespoons diced white onion

½ fresh jalapeño, seeded and minced, or pinch jalapeño powder

2 tablespoons chopped parsley flakes or cilantro, for garnish

DIRECTIONS:

1. In a bowl, using a fork, mash the avocado together with lime juice and salt. You can also use a mortar and pestle to achieve a smoother consistency.

2. Stir in the remaining ingredients. Feel free to use a food processor if you prefer a creamier guacamole.

3. Serve in a bowl and garnish with parsley flakes (or fresh cilantro) and enjoy as a dip or with any of your favorite dishes.

NOTE: Avocados tend to oxidize quickly, so this recipe is best enjoyed immediately! Refrigerate the leftovers for no more than one day in an airtight container for optimum freshness.

PER SERVING: 126 calories, 2 grams protein, 9 grams carbohydrates, 11 grams total fat

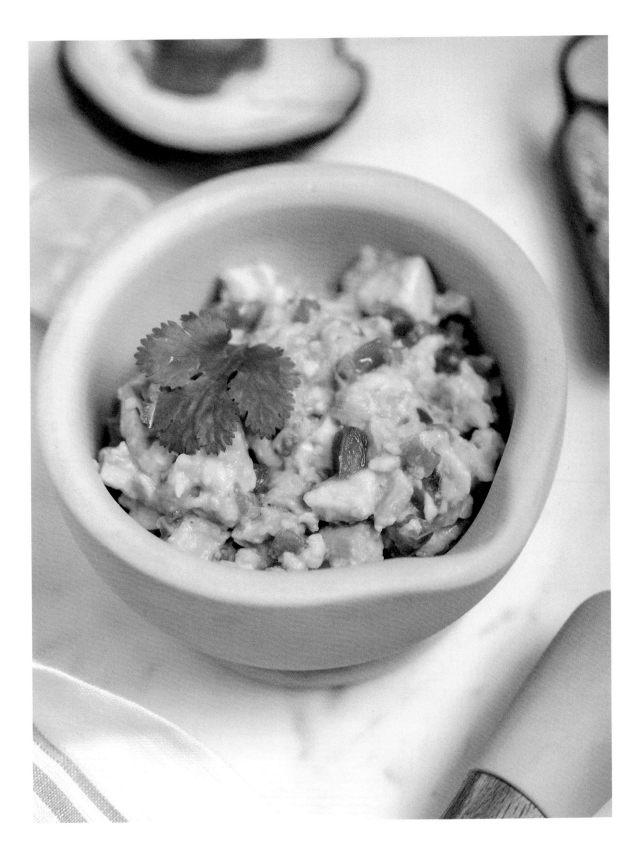

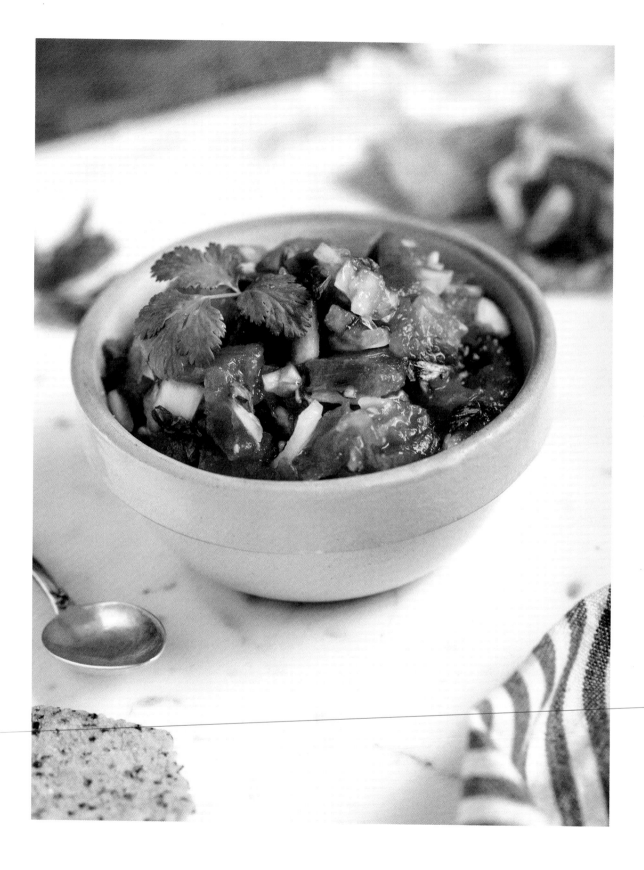

PICO DE GALLO

PREP TIME: 10 min

COOK TIME: 0 min

TOTAL TIME: 10 min

MAKES 4 SERVINGS

This Pico de Gallo can be enjoyed as a dip and as a garnish for many of our recipes, some of which include the Stuffed Bell Pepper Cups with Lentils & Avocado (see recipe on page 187), Black Bean Burrito Bowl (see recipe on page 200), and the Cuban Brown Rice Bowl (see recipe on page 203).

INGREDIENTS:

2 large tomatoes, diced (about 2 cups)

1 small white onion, finely diced (½ cup)

2 tablespoons parsley flakes, chopped, or cilantro, plus more for garnish

1 jalapeño, minced, lightly seeded

1 garlic clove, minced, or pinch of garlic powder (optional)

1 lime, juiced

¼ teaspoon sea salt, to taste

DIRECTIONS:

1. In a bowl, mix together all ingredients.

2. Place the Pico de Gallo in a serving bowl and garnish with parsley flakes or fresh cilantro and enjoy!

PER ½ CUP SERVING: 24 calories, 0 grams protein, 6 grams carbohydrates, 0 grams total fat

LIGHT

MASHED CAULIFLOWER

PREP TIME: 5 min

COOK TIME: 25 min

TOTAL TIME: 30 min

MAKES 4 SERVINGS

Move over, mashed potatoes. You have some competition. Cauliflower is an excellent source of vitamins C, K, and B_6, folate, fiber, and omega-3 fatty acids. In addition to a nutritional punch, this recipe has creamy goodness.

INGREDIENTS:

4 cups cauliflower florets (1 large head)

1 clove garlic, minced

2 tablespoons extra-virgin olive oil

sea salt, to taste

pinch of chives, diced, for garnish

PREPARATION:

1. Preheat oven to 450F and line a baking sheet with parchment paper.

2. Bring a large pot of salted water to a boil.

3. Add 3 cups of cauliflower florets to the pot and boil for 8–10 minutes or until tender.

4. Drain the florets and transfer them to a blender or food processor.

5. Add the garlic and 1 tablespoon of olive oil and puree until smooth. Taste and adjust seasoning, if necessary. Set aside while preparing the garnish.

6. To prepare the garnish, toss the remaining 1 cup of cauliflower florets with 1 tablespoon of olive oil and a pinch of sea salt. Bake the mixture on the parchment-lined sheet for 15 minutes or until slightly golden.

7. In a serving dish, spread the mashed cauliflower and garnish with the baked cauliflower florets and a pinch of chives, and enjoy!

PER SERVING: 114 calories, 4 grams protein, 11 grams carbohydrates, 8 grams total fat

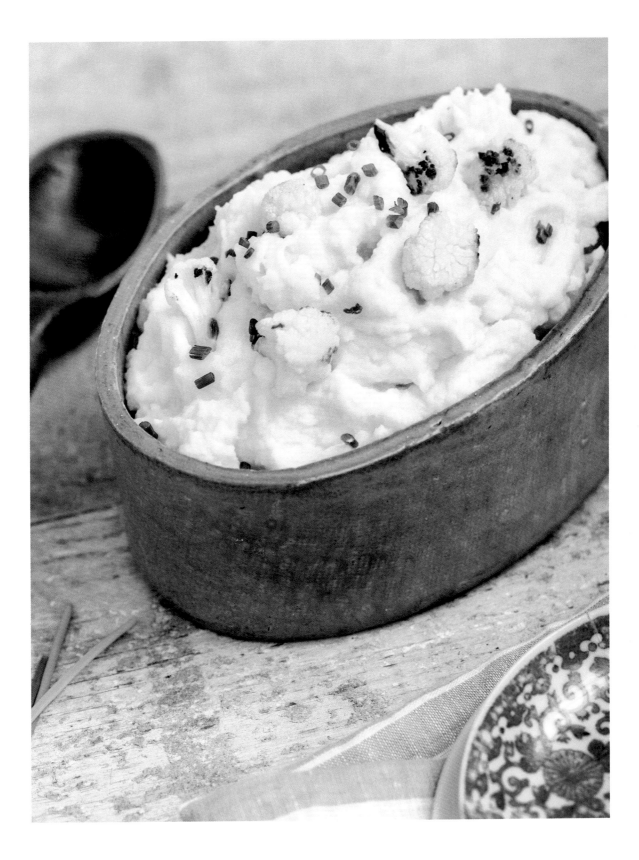

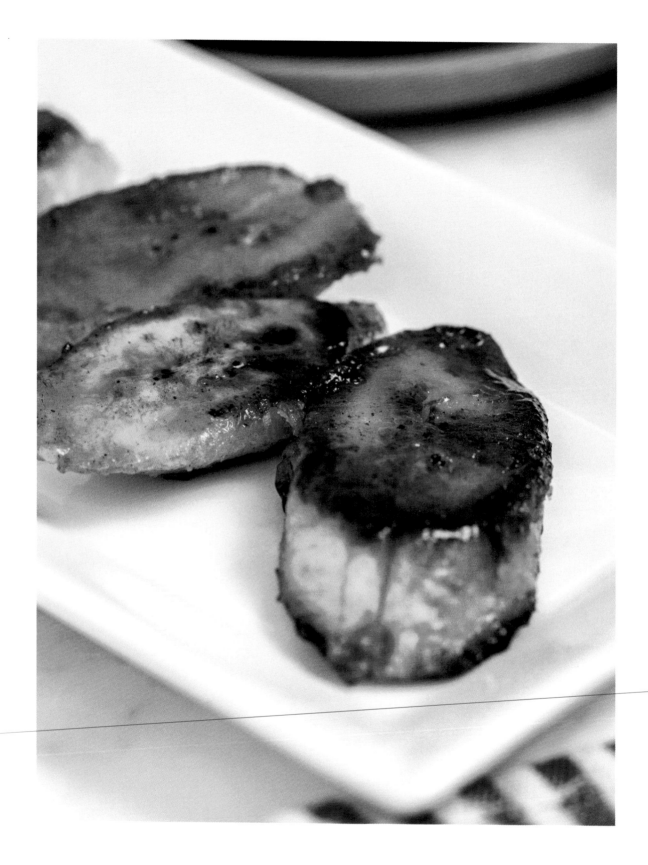

PLÁTANOS MADUROS (SWEET PLANTAINS), OVEN-BAKED

PREP TIME: 5 min

COOK TIME: 30 min

TOTAL TIME: 35 min

MAKES 4 SERVINGS

While I was growing up, there were a few things you could always find at our dinner table. One of them was plátanos maduros. Plantains are a member of the banana family. They're a great source of potassium and fiber, and they contain more vitamins A and C than their cousins. You'll love the delicious sweetness of these golden brown beauties. I could honestly have these every day for the rest of my life and not tire of them.

INGREDIENTS:

2 very ripe plantains, brownish or black and very tender to the touch

DIRECTIONS:

1. Preheat oven to 400F and line a baking sheet with parchment paper.

2. Cut off the ends of the plantains and draw a sharp knife along the peel, lengthwise, making 2 or 3 slits from one end to the other.

3. Carefully peel off the skin in sections.

4. Slice each plantain diagonally into ½-inch-thick oval slices. Or slice the plantains down the middle in half and then lengthwise to create 4 pieces.

5. Place the plantains on the baking sheet and bake for about 30 minutes.

6. When the plantains are soft and caramelized, remove from the oven and enjoy!

OPTIONAL:

▶ You can also cook the plantains in a large skillet that's lightly greased with coconut oil, over medium-high heat, for about 5 minutes on each side.

PER SERVING: 109 calories, 1 gram protein, 29 grams carbohydrates, 0 grams total fat

ROASTED BALSAMIC BRUSSELS SPROUTS

PREP TIME: 15 min
COOK TIME: 35 min
TOTAL TIME: 50 min

MAKES 4 SERVINGS

Here's another side that belongs on menus across the country. Brussels sprouts are full of flavor and rich in vitamins K, C, and B$_6$, folate, manganese, fiber, and potassium, which make a perfect accompaniment to any dish.

INGREDIENTS:

1 pound brussels sprouts

2 tablespoons canola oil

1 tablespoon balsamic vinegar

½ teaspoon sea salt or to taste

ground black pepper, to taste

pinch of rosemary

PREPARATION:

1. Preheat oven to 375F and line a baking sheet with parchment paper.

2. In a colander, rinse and drain the brussels sprouts.

3. Cut the stems, remove loose outer leaves, and slice the brussels sprouts into halves.

4. Place the brussels sprouts in a mixing bowl and toss with the oil, balsamic vinegar, salt, pepper, and rosemary. Allow the ingredients to marinate for a few minutes.

5. Place the mixture on the baking sheet and roast for about 30–35 minutes, tossing at least once for even browning.

6. Remove from the oven and enjoy!

PER SERVING: 112 calories, 4 grams protein, 10 grams carbohydrates, 7 grams total fat

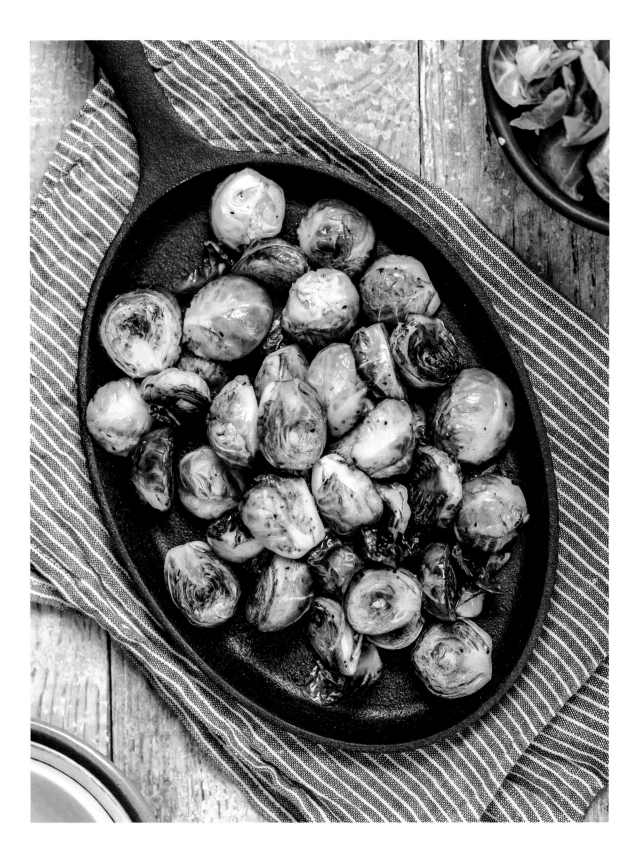

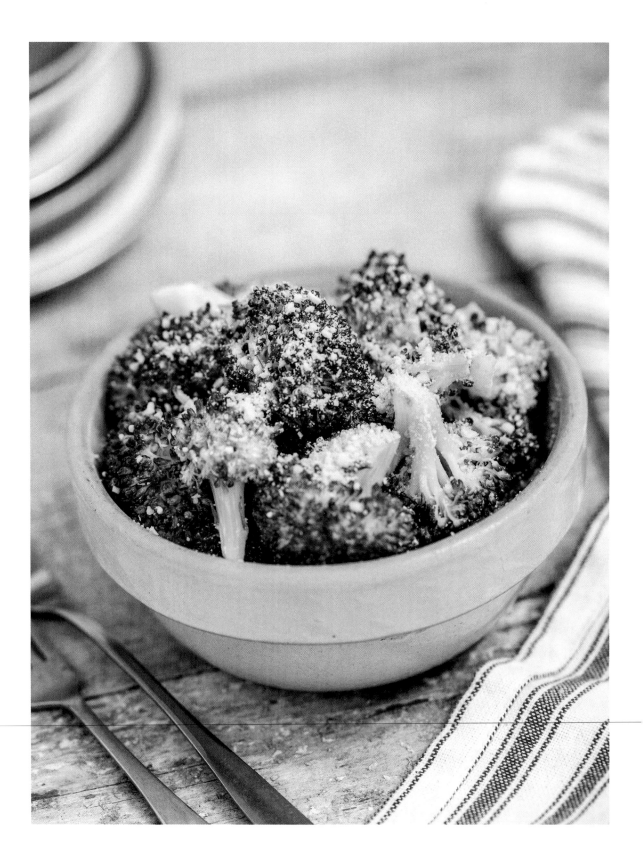

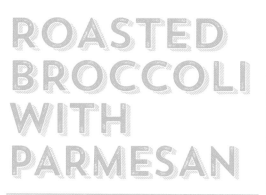

ROASTED BROCCOLI WITH PARMESAN

PREP TIME: 10 min

COOK TIME: 20 min

TOTAL TIME: 30 min

MAKES 4 SERVINGS

This is a simple way to introduce the bountiful nutritional benefits of broccoli to kids, in a dish they're sure to love.

INGREDIENTS:

2 large heads broccoli, cut into florets

2 tablespoons canola oil

¾ teaspoon sea salt or to taste

ground black pepper, to taste

2 tablespoons Parmesan Cheese (see recipe on page 340)

PREPARATION:

1. Preheat oven to 400F.

2. In a colander, rinse and drain the broccoli.

3. In a mixing bowl, toss together the broccoli with the oil, salt, and pepper.

4. Place the broccoli mixture on a sheet pan and roast for about 20 minutes until crisp yet tender.

5. Remove from the oven, immediately toss with Parmesan Cheese, and serve!

PER SERVING: 106 calories, 3 grams protein, 5 grams carbohydrates, 9 grams total fat

LIGHT

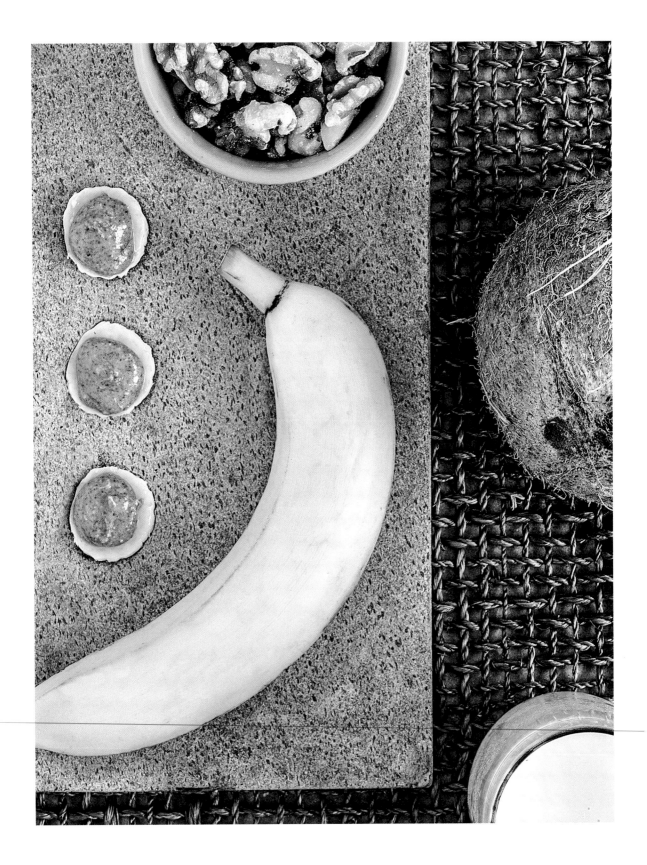

INDULGENT SNACKS AND SIDES

(150 CALORIES OR MORE)

INDULGENT

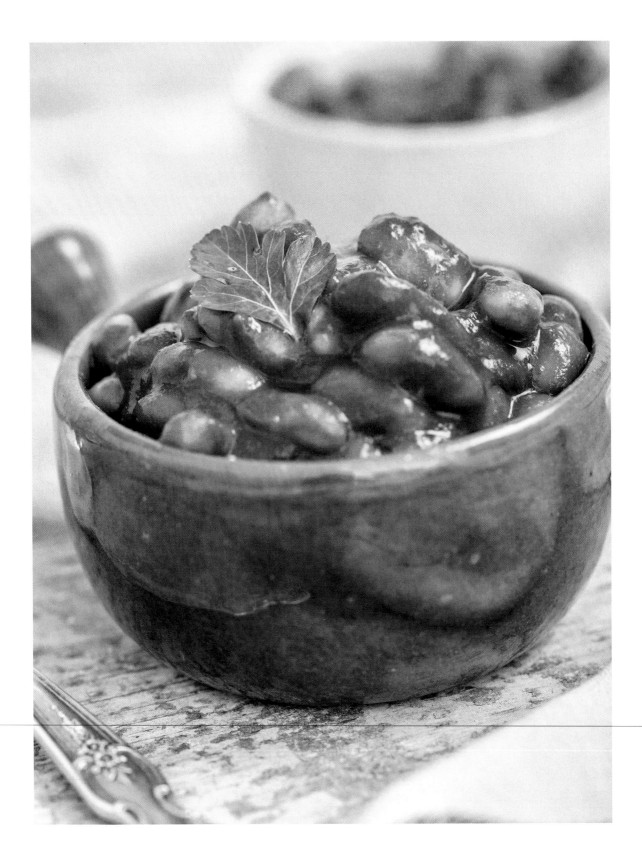

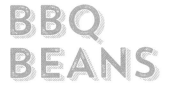
BBQ BEANS

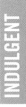

PREP TIME: 10 min

COOK TIME: 2 hrs

TOTAL TIME: 2 hrs 10 min

MAKES 4 SERVINGS

Beans are a rich source of iron, potassium, protein, folate, fiber, vitamins, and minerals. This is a side that can easily be a main dish. We love these topped with avocados!

INGREDIENTS:

1 cup Great Northern beans, uncooked, soaked overnight in 3 cups of water

2½ cups water

1 cup BBQ Sauce (see recipe on page 312)

1 teaspoon maple syrup

pinch of sea salt

PREPARATION:

1. Rinse and drain the beans.

2. Add the beans and 2½ cups of water to a pot and bring to a boil.

3. Reduce heat to medium-low and cook the beans for about 2 hours, adding the BBQ Sauce, maple syrup, and salt halfway through cooking. Add water and adjust seasoning, if necessary.

4. Once the beans are tender, serve them and enjoy!

TIP: Store leftovers in an airtight container in the refrigerator for no more than a few days.

PER SERVING: 194 calories, 11 grams protein, 37 grams carbohydrates, 1 gram total fat

CHOCOLATE CHIA PUDDING

PREP TIME: 5 min

COOK TIME: 0 min

TOTAL TIME: 5 min (does not include refrigeration time)

MAKES 2 SERVINGS

Chia seeds are a great source of heart-healthy omega-3 fatty acids, and this pudding is loaded with heart-health benefits plus an extra kick of protein.

INGREDIENTS:

3 tablespoons chia seeds

1 cup sweetened vanilla almond milk (or other nondairy alternative)

1 scoop 22 Days Chocolate Plant-Protein Powder

2 teaspoons of cacao powder (or cocoa powder)

1 tablespoon maple syrup (add 1 more if prefer sweeter)

1 tablespoon vegan chocolate chips, for sprinkling

PREPARATION:

1. In a blender, place all the ingredients except the chocolate chips and blend until smooth. Taste and adjust sweetness if necessary.

2. Pour the pudding mixture into two serving cups and refrigerate for about 30 minutes or longer to allow the mixture to thicken and chill.

3. Serve cold with a sprinkling of chocolate chips and enjoy!

PER SERVING: 386 calories, 23 grams protein, 44 grams carbohydrates, 16 grams total fat

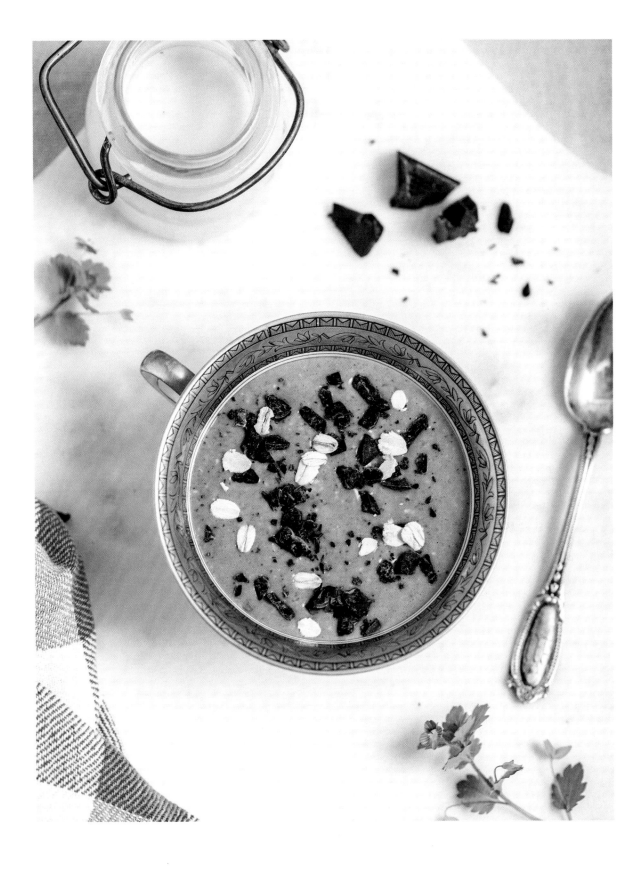

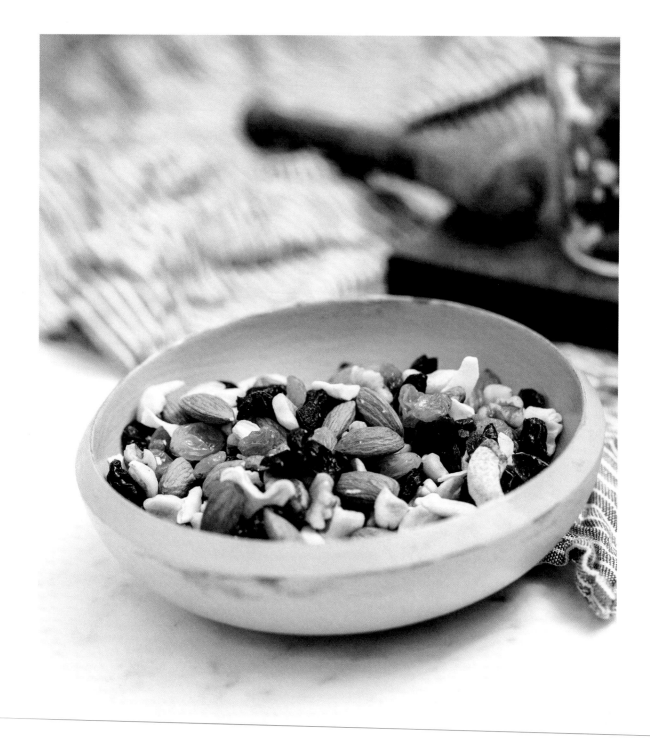
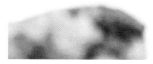

SUPERFOOD TRAIL MIX

PREP TIME: 5 min

COOK TIME: 0 min

TOTAL TIME: 5 min

MAKES 4 SERVINGS

This superfood trail mix is not only a great source of protein and fiber, but it is also packed with many beneficial vitamins and antioxidants. It makes a great addition for breakfast. Or simply enjoy the trail mix as a healthy and energizing snack.

INGREDIENTS:

½ cup raw almonds

½ cup raw cashews

¼ cup raw walnuts

¼ cup golden berries

¼ cup raisins

2 tablespoons dried cranberries

1 tablespoon unsweetened coconut flakes

DIRECTIONS:

1. In a bowl, mix all the ingredients together.

2. Serve and enjoy!

TIP: Store in a mason jar.

PER SERVING: 348 calories, 9 grams protein, 33 grams carbohydrates, 22 grams total fat

CRISPY LENTILS

PREP TIME: 10 min

COOK TIME: 45 min

TOTAL TIME: 55 min

MAKES 2 SERVINGS

Lentils are an incredibly powerful protein source and one of the best alkaline protein sources in the world. Our family loves the way they taste, so we have fun creating all kinds of recipes with them. Here's one you won't see often.

INGREDIENTS:

¾ cup uncooked lentils or 1 15-ounce can, drained and rinsed

½ tablespoon extra-virgin olive oil

½ teaspoon garlic powder

sea salt, to taste

ground black pepper, to taste

PREPARATION:

1. Rinse lentils and place them in a pot with water (about 2 inches above the lentils) and bring to a boil.

2. Reduce the heat to a simmer and cook for about 20 minutes, stirring occasionally.

3. Preheat oven to 375F and line a baking sheet with parchment paper.

4. Once the lentils are tender, drain them in a colander and pat them dry to remove excess moisture.

5. Place the lentils in a bowl and toss together with the oil, garlic powder, sea salt, and pepper.

6. Spread the lentils on the baking sheet and bake for 24 to 26 minutes or until crispy. Stir once or twice during the cooking time to prevent burning.

7. Let the lentils cool and enjoy!

TIP: Once completely cool, the lentils can be stored in an airtight container or a mason jar. The lentils are best if eaten within a few days.

PER SERVING: 191 calories, 12 grams protein, 29 grams carbohydrates, 3 grams total fat

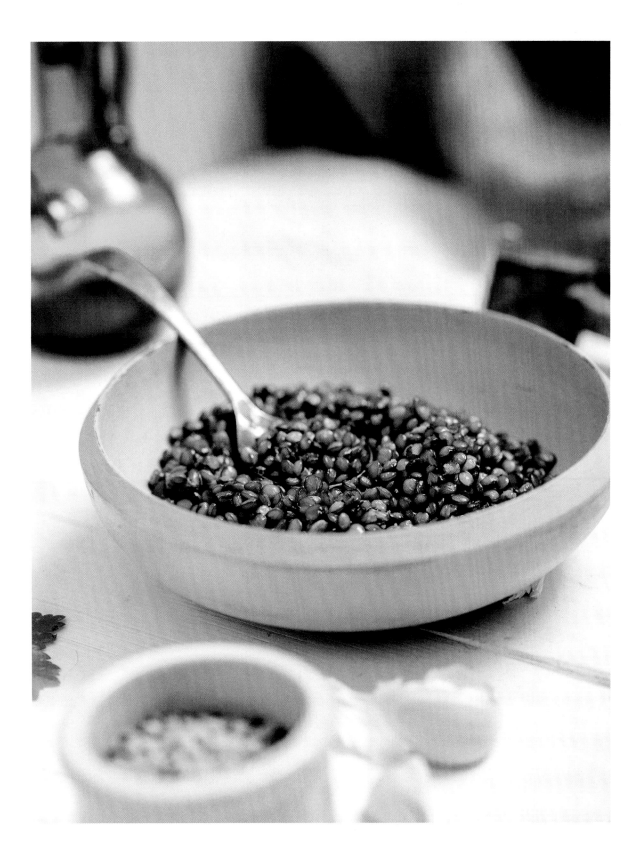

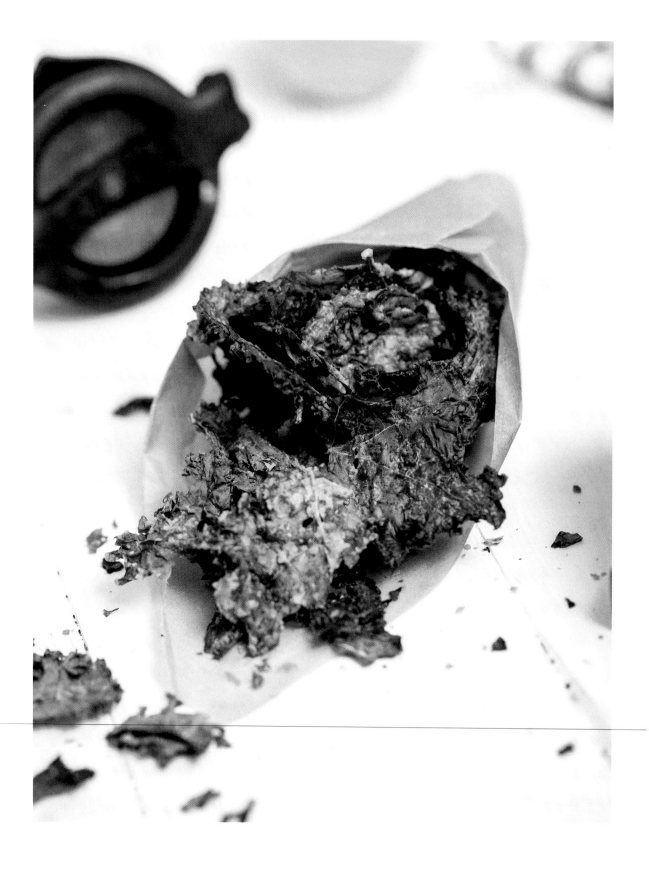

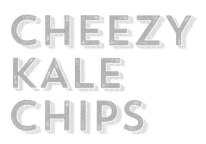

CHEEZY KALE CHIPS

PREP TIME: 10 min

COOK TIME: 35 min

TOTAL TIME: 45 min (doesn't include cashew soak time)

MAKES 4 SERVINGS

I fell in love with kale chips after buying them at a local grocer but loved them even more once we created a recipe for them at home. We usually opt for the dehydrator as our preferred method of preparing them, but our kids love them any way we serve them.

INGREDIENTS:

1 large bunch curly kale, destemmed

1 cup raw cashews, presoaked in warm water for 30 minutes

1 small red bell pepper, washed, seeded, and chopped

2 tablespoons nutritional yeast

1 lemon, juiced

1 teaspoon milled chia seeds

½–¾ teaspoon sea salt or to taste

¼ cup water

PREPARATION:

1. Preheat oven to 300F and line a baking sheet with parchment paper. Might have to use two baking sheets.

2. Wash the kale leaves and let them thoroughly dry.

3. Rinse and drain the cashews and transfer them to a food processor or blender. Add the pepper, nutritional yeast, lemon juice, chia, salt, and water. Blend until smooth.

4. Tear the washed and dried kale into pieces with your hands and transfer it to a mixing bowl.

5. Toss the kale together with the sauce and massage well with your hands. Place the kale on the baking sheet, making sure the pieces are spread out in a single layer and not overlapping for optimum crispness.

6. Bake for about 30–35 minutes, flipping the kale halfway through cooking.

7. If you prefer to use a dehydrator, set it for about 12 hours at 110F. The kale chips are ready when crisp.

TIP: If there are any leftovers, feel free to use as a garnish for Kale-Yeah Soup (see recipe on page 142).

PER SERVING: 256 calories, 10 grams protein, 21 grams carbohydrates, 17 grams total fat

CHEESY CAULIFLOWER

PREP TIME: 5 min

COOK TIME: 20 min

TOTAL TIME: 25 min (does not include Mozzarella Cheese recipe cook time)

MAKES 4 SERVINGS

Veggies don't have to be boring to be nutritious. This is a dish that I wish was on every menu across the country: a perfect blend of flavor, texture, and nutritional benefits!

INGREDIENTS:

1 large head cauliflower

1 tablespoon ground paprika

½ lime, juiced

¼–½ teaspoon sea salt or to taste

4 tablespoons Mozzarella Cheese (see recipe on page 336)

chives, for garnish

PREPARATION:

1. Preheat oven to 450F.

2. Wash and cut the cauliflower into small florets.

3. In a bowl, mix the paprika, lime juice, and sea salt together.

4. Fold in the cauliflower florets.

5. Scoop the mixture into 4 portion-size oven-safe baking dishes or 1 large baking dish. Top with cheese.

6. Bake for about 15–20 minutes or until golden.

7. Garnish with chives and enjoy!

PER SERVING: 186 calories, 8 grams protein, 21 grams carbohydrates, 10 grams total fat

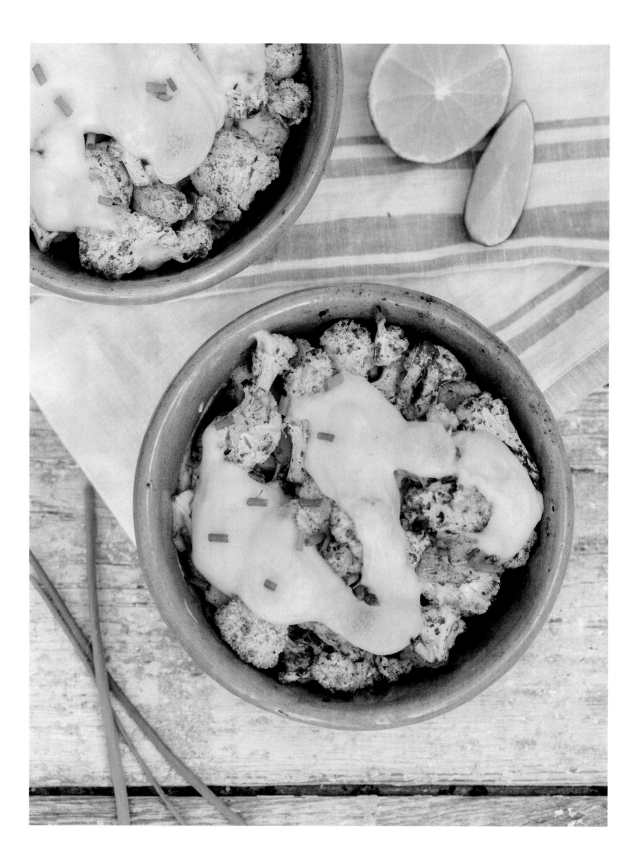

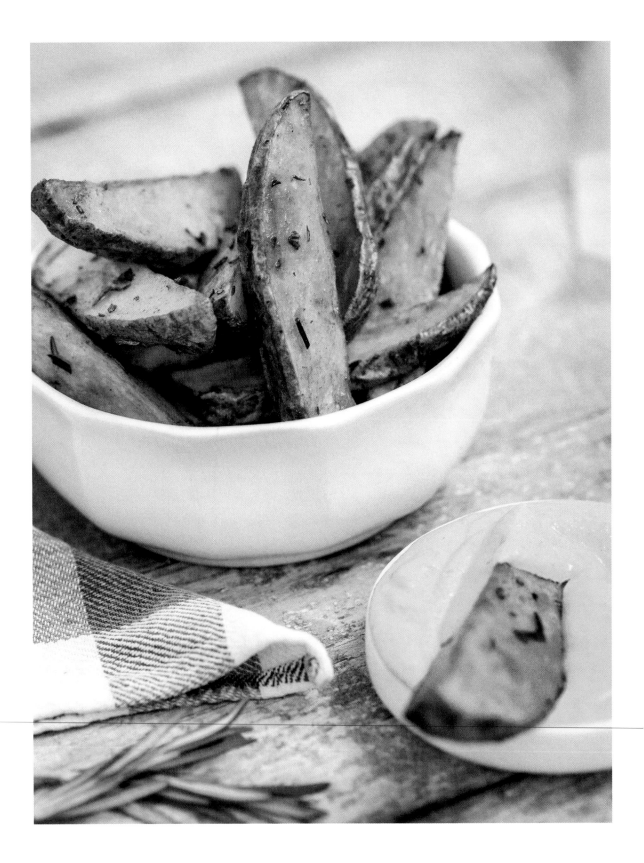

OVEN-BAKED POTATO FRIES WITH NACHO CHEESE

PREP TIME: 15 min

COOK TIME: 40 min

TOTAL TIME: 55 min

MAKES 4 SERVINGS

We all love French fries but not the feelings that accompany them. This is a delicious alternative bursting with flavor that will nourish and satisfy you while you practice a habit of making healthier selections.

INGREDIENTS:

4 medium Yukon gold potatoes

2 tablespoons olive oil

1 teaspoon ground cumin

1 teaspoon ground smoked paprika

pinch of rosemary

pinch of sea salt

Nacho Cheese (see recipe on page 339)

PREPARATION:

1. Preheat oven to 350F and line a baking sheet with parchment paper.

2. Thoroughly wash the potatoes, then slice them into wedges.

3. In a bowl, toss the potato wedges with the remaining ingredients except the Nacho Cheese.

4. Place the potatoes in the oven and bake for about 40 minutes.

5. Remove the potatoes from the oven, drizzle them with Nacho Cheese and enjoy!

PER SERVING: 277 calories, 6 grams protein, 41 grams carbohydrates, 11 grams total fat

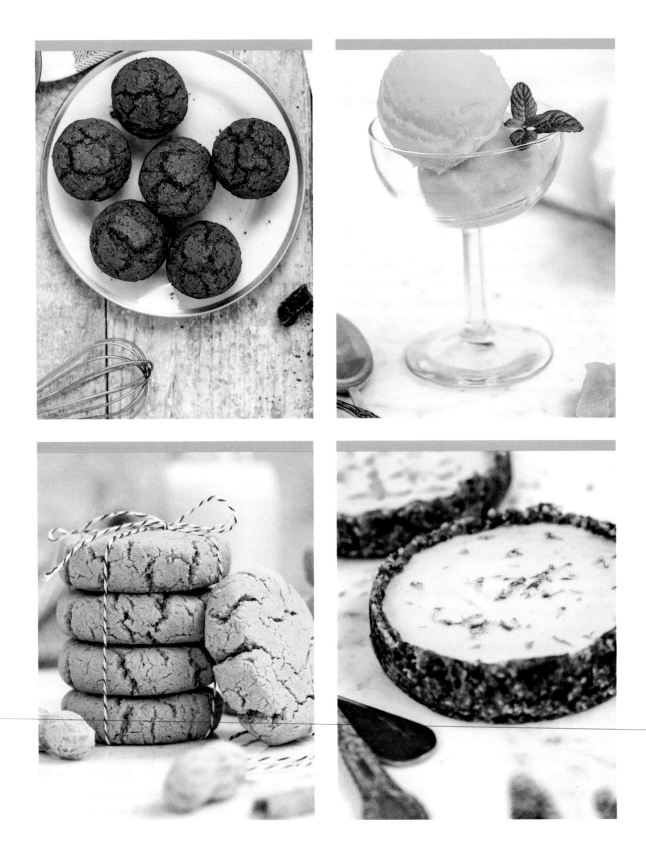

DESSERTS

EATING PLANT-BASED DOESN'T MEAN giving up on the finer things in life, like desserts. Sweet treats that tempt your palate don't have to ruin your waistline or your figure. Keep your mood sweet while you delight your family, your guests, and yourself with our Brownie Bites, Chocolate Chip Cookies or my recent favorite, Plátanos Maduros à la Mode.

In my house, we often have fruit for dessert, because the sweetness of berries and apples and pears and mangoes is a treat we all relish. But sometimes, when we really feel like celebrating, my beautiful wife, Marilyn, will surprise us by whipping up her famous Maple Pecan Bliss Balls or Raw Key Lime Pie. (Yes, we've included the recipes here for you.)

Our desserts are wonderful additions to a special meal, as a hostess gift or at any party. On a daily basis, you can make room for a refreshing Watermelon Slush or melt-in-your-mouth Coconut Ice Cream; just keep an eye on calorie counts and portion sizes. True enjoyment is when your indulgences are a balanced part of your meal plan, and there's nothing more decadent than losing weight and eating cake too.

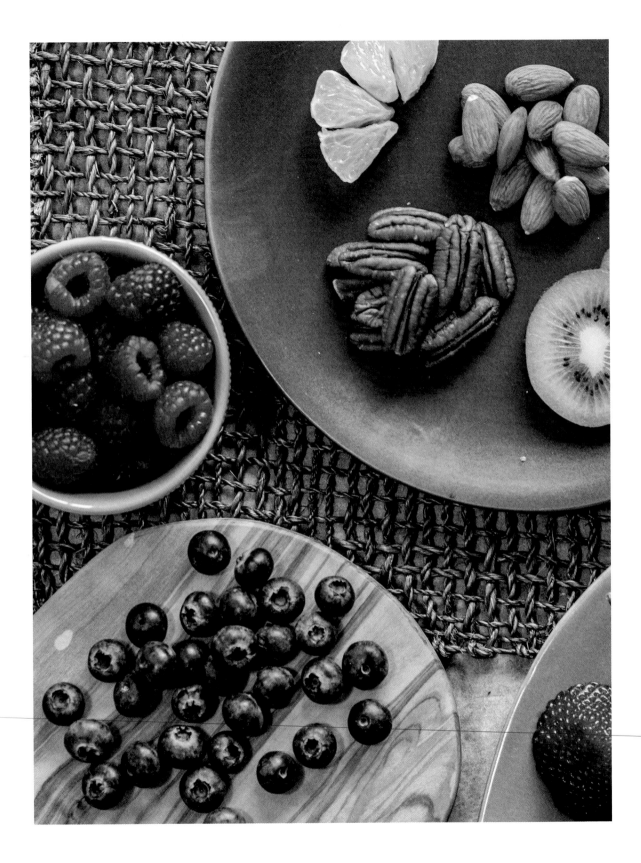

LIGHT DESSERTS

(UNDER 150 CALORIES)

LIGHT

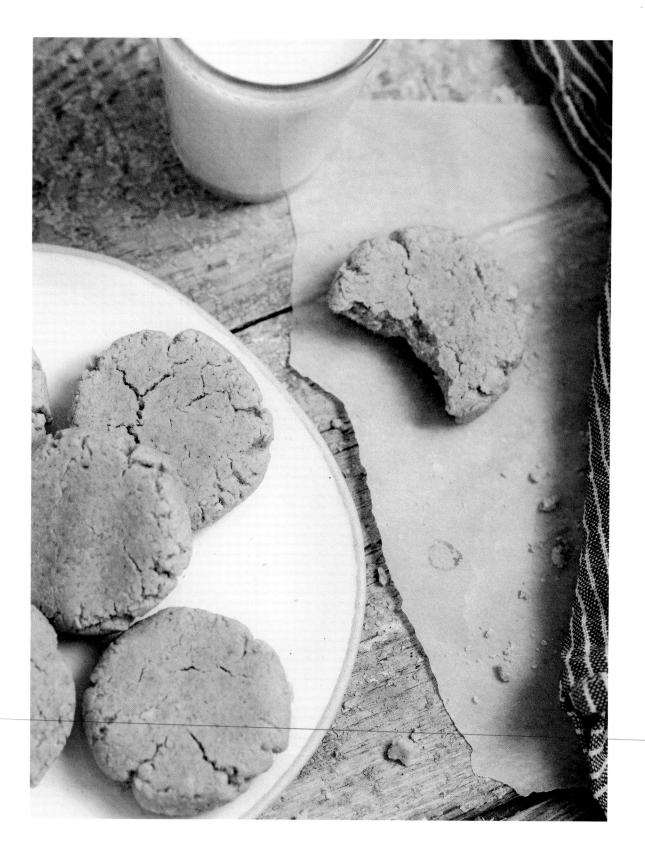

ALMOND OAT COOKIES

▶ **NO OIL** ▶ **REFINED SUGAR-FREE**

PREP TIME: 5 min

COOK TIME: 10 min

TOTAL TIME: 15 min

MAKES 18 COOKIES

These almond cookies are made without the use of added oil and can be easily made without too much time in the kitchen, which means there will be less cleanup required.

INGREDIENTS:

1 cup almond flour

1 cup gluten-free oat flour

1 teaspoon baking powder

4 tablespoons sweetened vanilla almond milk

4 tablespoons maple syrup

PREPARATION:

1. Preheat oven to 350F. Line a baking sheet with parchment paper.

2. In a bowl, mix together the almond flour, oat flour, and baking powder.

3. In another bowl, mix together the almond milk and maple syrup.

4. Thoroughly combine the dry ingredients with the wet, using your hands if necessary.

5. Form the dough into balls, press into your desired cookie shape, and place on the baking sheet at least one inch apart.

6. Bake for 10–12 minutes (or 12–14 minutes for a crispier cookie).

7. Let cool and enjoy!

PER SERVING: 70 calories, 2 grams protein, 9 grams carbohydrates, 3 grams total fat

BROWNIE BITES

PREP TIME: 5 min

COOK TIME: 18 min

TOTAL TIME: 23 min

MAKES 12 BITES

Warning: If you have children, you may want to start with a couple of batches at once if you plan to try one yourself. Brownies have never been so delicious.

INGREDIENTS:

½ cup oat flour

¼ cup tapioca flour

2 tablespoons flax meal

1 tablespoon almond flour

2 tablespoons raw cane sugar

2 tablespoons cocoa powder

½ teaspoon baking soda

4 tablespoons vanilla almond milk

3 tablespoons maple syrup

2 tablespoons applesauce

1 teaspoon apple cider vinegar

PREPARATION:

1. Preheat oven to 350F. Lightly grease a mini-muffin pan or line with paper liners.

2. In a bowl, whisk together the dry ingredients.

3. In another bowl, mix together the wet ingredients.

4. Pour the wet ingredients over the dry and mix until well combined.

5. Pour the batter into the muffin pan.

6. Bake for 16–18 minutes. Remove the brownies from the oven and let cool before transferring them to a wire rack.

TIP: Leftovers can be stored at room temperature in an airtight container for up to a few days, in the refrigerator for up to 1 week, or in the freezer, in freezer bags layered with parchment paper, for up to a few months.

PER SERVING: 69 calories, 2 grams protein, 13 grams carbohydrates, 1 gram total fat

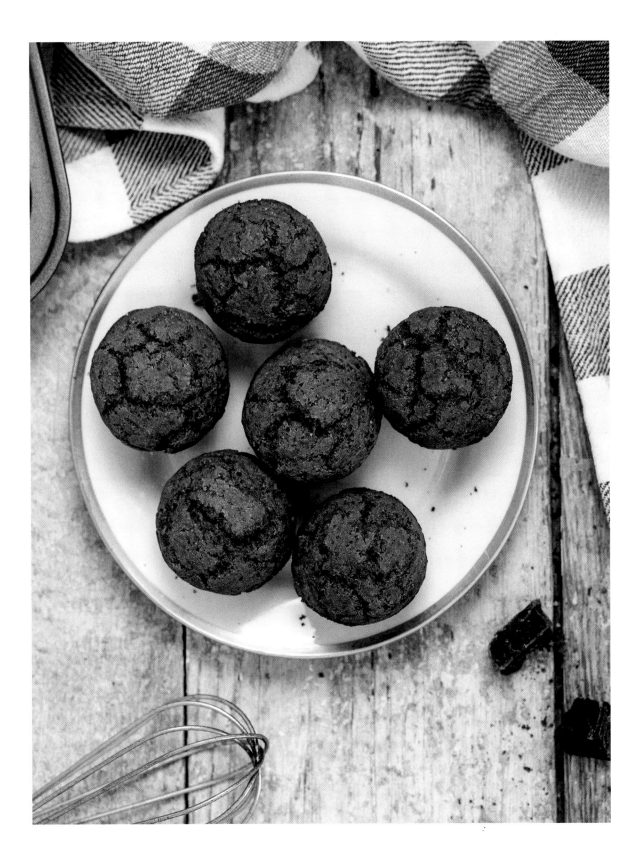

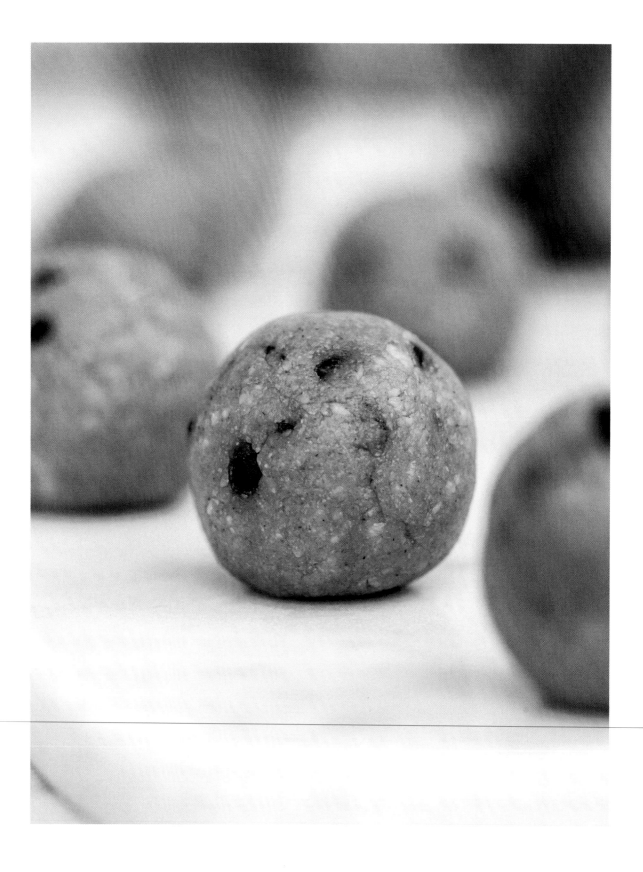

CHOCOLATE CHIP COOKIE DOUGH BLISS BALLS

PREP TIME: 15 min

COOK TIME: 0 min

TOTAL TIME: 15 min

MAKES 12 BALLS

Once you've made these, you may decide to keep some in the fridge all the time as a quick pick-me-up. Our boys love these as an after-school snack.

INGREDIENTS:

½ cup raw cashews

½ cup gluten-free oat flour

2 tablespoons water

3 tablespoons maple syrup or coconut nectar

2 tablespoons mini dark chocolate chips

PREPARATION:

1. In a food processor, add the cashews and pulse until a flourlike consistency is reached.

2. Add the oat flour, water, and maple syrup and blend together until well combined.

3. Scoop the mixture into a bowl and fold in the chocolate chips.

4. Divide the mixture into tablespoon-sized balls and chill (optional).

TIP: Leftovers can be refrigerated in an airtight container for up to 1 week.

PER SERVING: 81 calories, 2 grams protein, 10 grams carbohydrates, 4 grams total fat

CHOCOLATE CHIP COOKIES

▶ **NUT-FREE** ▶ **GLUTEN-FREE**

PREP TIME: 10 min

COOK TIME: 12 min

TOTAL TIME: 22 min

MAKES 20 COOKIES

These are a simple and delicious classic, made without nuts, gluten, or refined sugar. They're low in fat, light in calories, and full of flavor.

INGREDIENTS:

1 cup gluten-free oat flour

1 cup brown rice flour

½ cup tapioca flour

½ cup organic coconut palm sugar

1 tablespoon milled golden flaxseed

½ teaspoon baking powder

½ teaspoon baking soda

¼ cup sweetened vanilla almond milk

2 tablespoons maple syrup

3 tablespoons melted coconut oil

½ teaspoon vanilla extract

¼ cup chocolate chips

PREPARATION:

1. Preheat oven to 350F. Line a cookie sheet with parchment paper.

2. In a mixing bowl, stir together the dry ingredients except for the chocolate chips.

3. In a separate bowl, mix together the wet ingredients. Make sure all wet ingredients are at room temperature, to prevent the coconut oil from hardening.

4. Mix the wet ingredients into the dry ingredients until well combined. Then fold in the chocolate chips.

5. Refrigerate the dough for about 15 to 20 minutes so that it can slightly harden, making it easier to mold into cookie shapes.

6. Remove the dough from the refrigerator and scoop out a heaping tablespoon of dough onto the parchment paper. Shape dough with your hands and place cookies 1½ inches apart.

7. Bake for 10–12 minutes (or 12–14 minutes if you prefer a crispier texture). Let the cookies cool before carefully transferring them to a cooling rack. They will harden as they cool.

TIP: Store leftover cookies in an airtight container for up to a few days, in the refrigerator for up to 1 week, or in the freezer for up to 2 months.

PER SERVING: 116 calories, 20 grams carbohydrates, 3 grams total fat

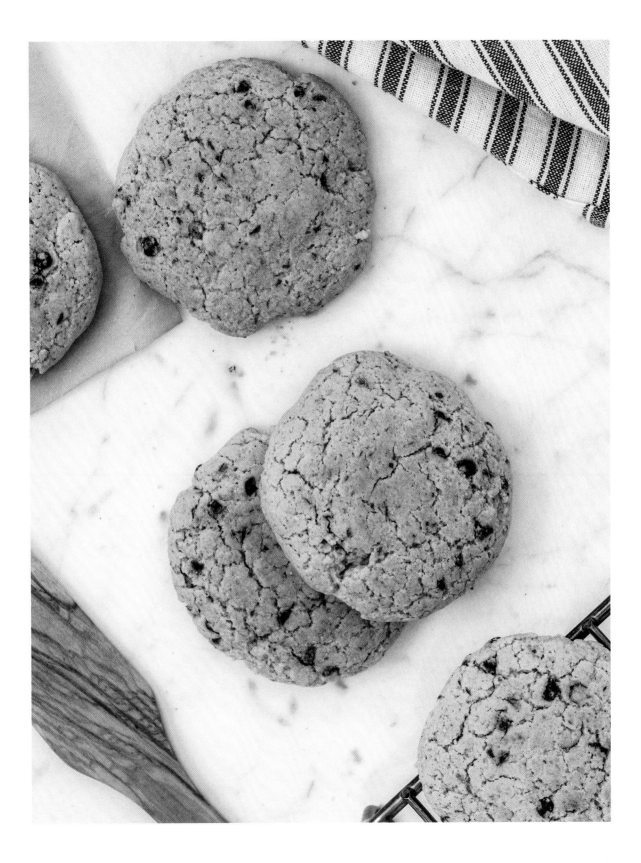

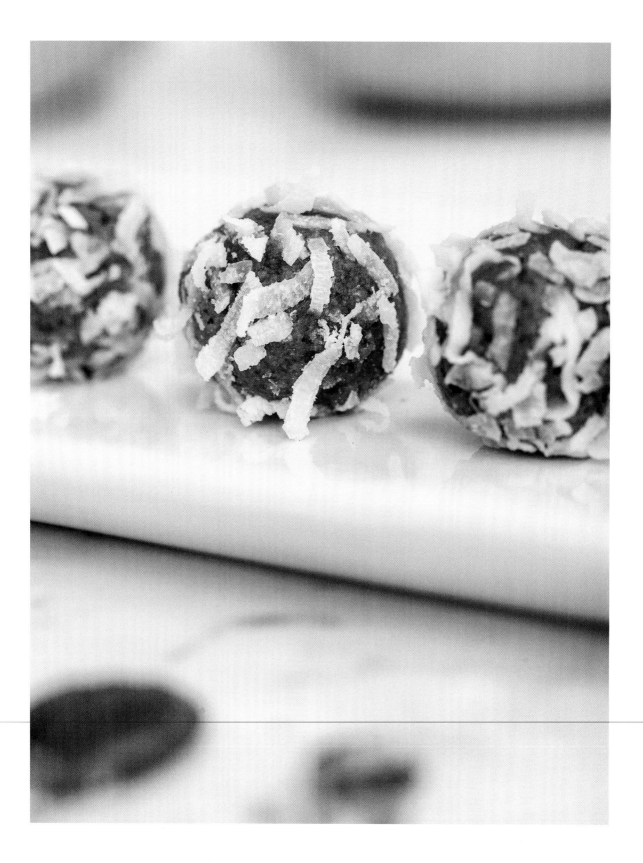

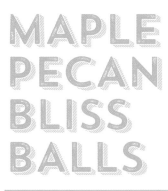

MAPLE PECAN BLISS BALLS

PREP TIME: 20 min

COOK TIME: 0 min

TOTAL TIME: 20 min

MAKES 16 BALLS

These Maple Pecan Bliss Balls are as simple as they are delicious! They make heart-healthy treats your whole family will enjoy.

INGREDIENTS:

½ cup gluten-free oat flour

½ cup pecan meal

2 tablespoons water

2 tablespoons maple syrup or coconut nectar

1 teaspoon sunflower seed butter

1 teaspoon milled flaxseed

1 cup shredded coconut, for coating

PREPARATION:

1. Mix all the ingredients together, except for the shredded coconut.

2. Divide the mixture into tablespoon-size balls.

3. Roll the balls in shredded coconut and enjoy!

TIP: Leftovers can be refrigerated in an airtight container for about 1 week.

PER SERVING: 54 calories, 1 gram protein, 5 grams carbohydrates, 3 grams total fat

WATERMELON SLUSH

PREP TIME: 10 min
COOK TIME: 0 min
TOTAL TIME: 10 min

2 SERVINGS

The only thing more refreshing than fresh watermelon may be Watermelon Slush. This is a summer favorite for kids. Watermelon is a rich source of vitamins A, B_6, and C, potassium, lycopene, and antioxidants, which makes for a perfect cooling treat.

INGREDIENTS:

4 cups seedless watermelon

4 tablespoons lemon juice

1 tablespoon maple syrup

lemon slices, for garnish

PREPARATION:

1. Freeze 3 cups of watermelon in freezer bags for at least 6 hours or overnight.

2. In a blender or food processor, place the remaining 1 cup (nonfrozen) watermelon. Add the frozen watermelon, lemon juice, and maple syrup. Blend the ingredients, scraping down the sides, until the mixture has reached a slushlike consistency.

3. Garnish with a slice of lemon and enjoy!

PER SERVING: 124 calories, 2 grams protein, 32 grams carbohydrates, 1 gram total fat

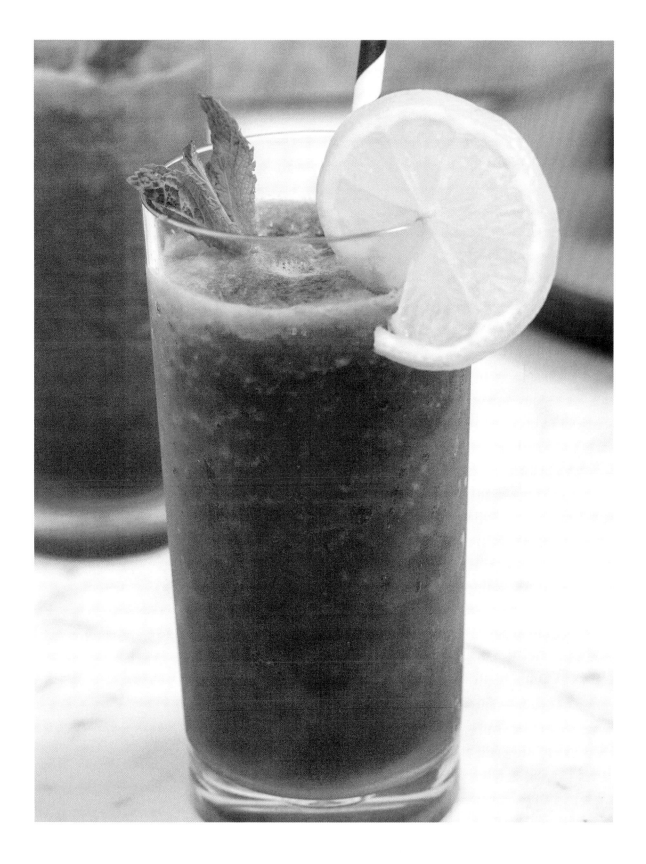

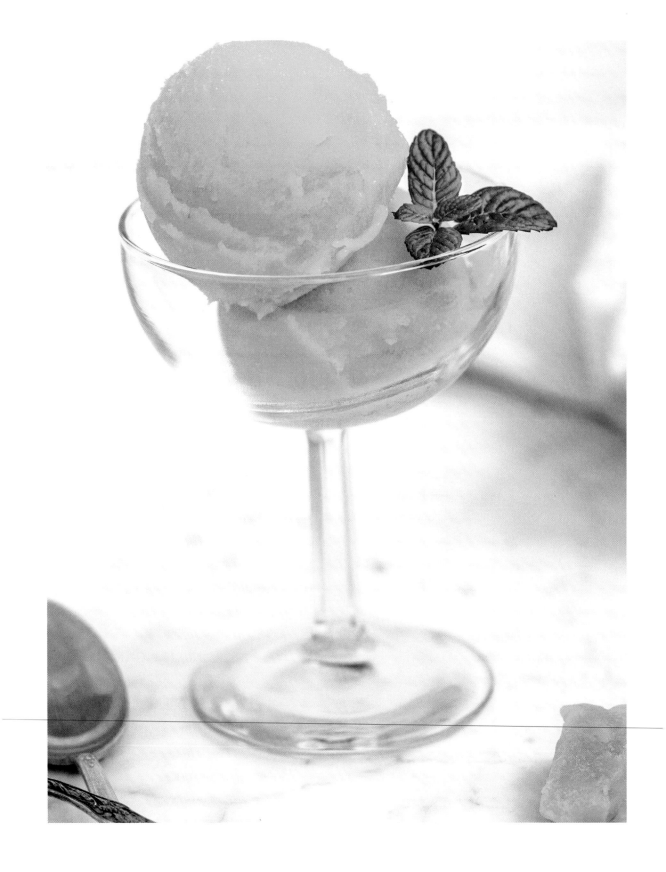

MANGO SORBET

PREP TIME: 10 min

COOK TIME: 0 min

TOTAL TIME: 10 min

MAKES 4 SERVINGS

This is a light dessert that's also rich in vitamins C and A and folate. It's the perfect refresher on a hot summer day.

INGREDIENTS:

4 cups frozen mango chunks

1 cup coconut water

¼ cup freshly squeezed orange juice

PREPARATION:

1. In a blender or food processor, blend all the ingredients together, scraping down the sides, until smooth.

2. Serve immediately or scoop the sorbet into a freezer-safe container or bread pan, and freeze for a couple of hours to harden.

3. When ready to enjoy, remove the sorbet from the freezer and let sit at room temperature for about 15 minutes to soften before serving.

4. Scoop sorbet into a bowl and enjoy!

PER SERVING: 117 calories, 2 grams protein, 29 grams carbohydrates, 1 gram total fat

ALMOND PULP COOKIES

PREP TIME: 5 min

COOK TIME: 10 min

TOTAL TIME: 15 min (does not include almond pulp prep)

MAKES 10 COOKIES

Here's a great way to use the almond pulp that will be left when you make almond milk at home. These cookies are delicious and easy to make.

INGREDIENTS:

1 cup almond pulp from Homemade Vanilla Almond Milk (see recipe on page 332)

1 cup gluten-free oat flour

¼ cup maple syrup

1 tablespoon coconut oil

¾ teaspoon baking powder

PREPARATION:

1. Preheat oven to 350F. Line a baking sheet with parchment paper.

2. In a bowl, thoroughly mix together all the ingredients.

3. Form the dough into balls, then into cookie shapes, and place them on the lined baking sheet.

4. Bake the cookies for about 10 minutes (for softer cookies) or for 15 minutes (if you prefer crispier cookies).

5. Let cool and enjoy!

PER SERVING: 137 calories, 4 grams protein, 18 grams carbohydrates, 6 grams total fat

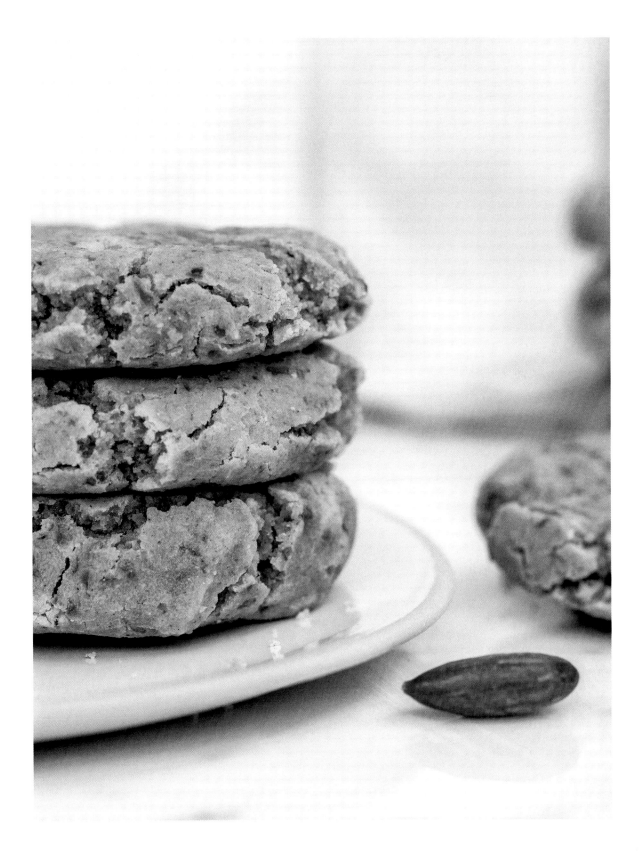

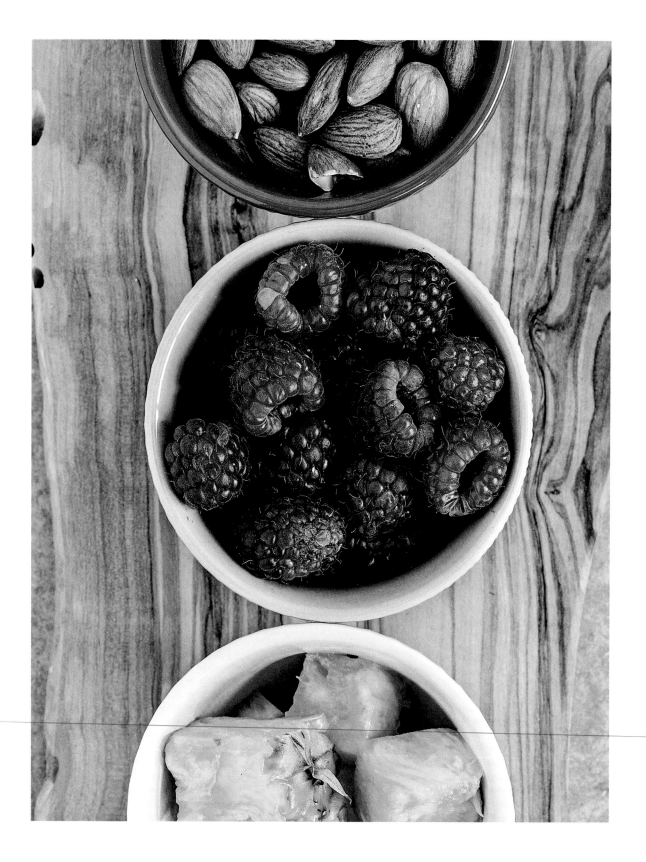

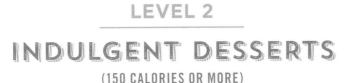

LEVEL 2

INDULGENT DESSERTS

(150 CALORIES OR MORE)

Peanut Butter Cookies 296

Banana Soft Serve with Date
Caramel Sauce 299

Coconut Ice Cream 300

Plátanos Maduros (Sweet Plantains)
à la Mode   303

Raw Key Lime Pie 304

INDULGENT

PEANUT BUTTER COOKIES

PREP TIME: 10 min

COOK TIME: 10 min

TOTAL TIME: 20 min

MAKES 12 COOKIES

While I was growing up, my favorite cookies were always peanut butter. This is an improvement on an old classic. Made without the usual butter and oil, these peanut butter cookies are better than the original.

INGREDIENTS:

1½ cups gluten-free oat flour

1 cup brown rice flour

4 tablespoons maple sugar

1 teaspoon baking soda

pinch of salt

5 tablespoons peanut butter

4 tablespoons sweetened vanilla almond milk

4 tablespoons maple syrup

1 teaspoon vanilla extract

2 tablespoons applesauce

PREPARATION:

1. Preheat oven to 350 F. Line a cookie sheet with parchment paper.

2. In a bowl, mix together the dry ingredients.

3. In another bowl, mix together the wet ingredients.

4. Thoroughly combine the dry ingredients with the wet.

5. Form the dough into balls, shape into desired cookie shape, and place them on the cookie sheet.

6. Bake for about 10–12 minutes. Cool and enjoy.

PER SERVING: 178 calories, 5 grams protein, 29 grams carbohydrates, 5 grams total fat

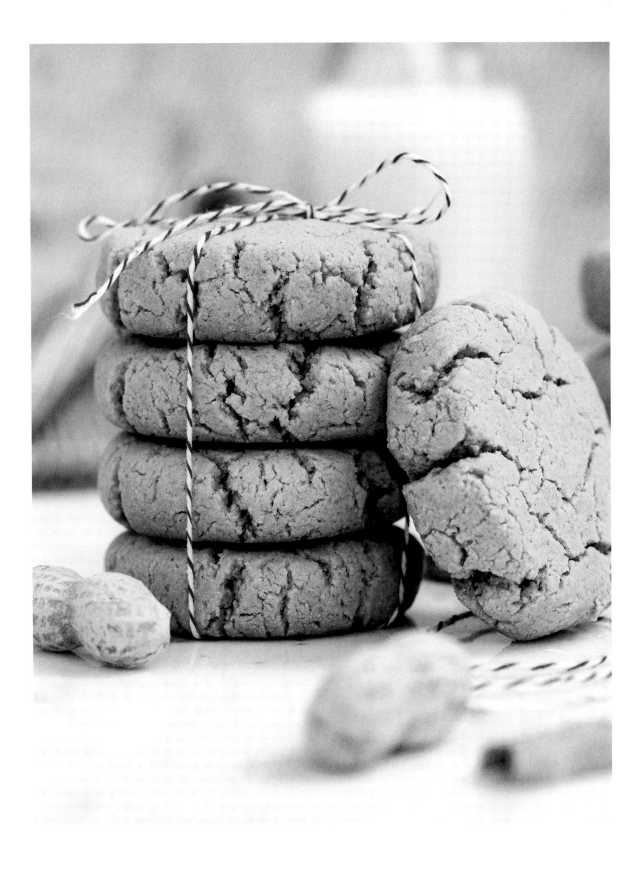

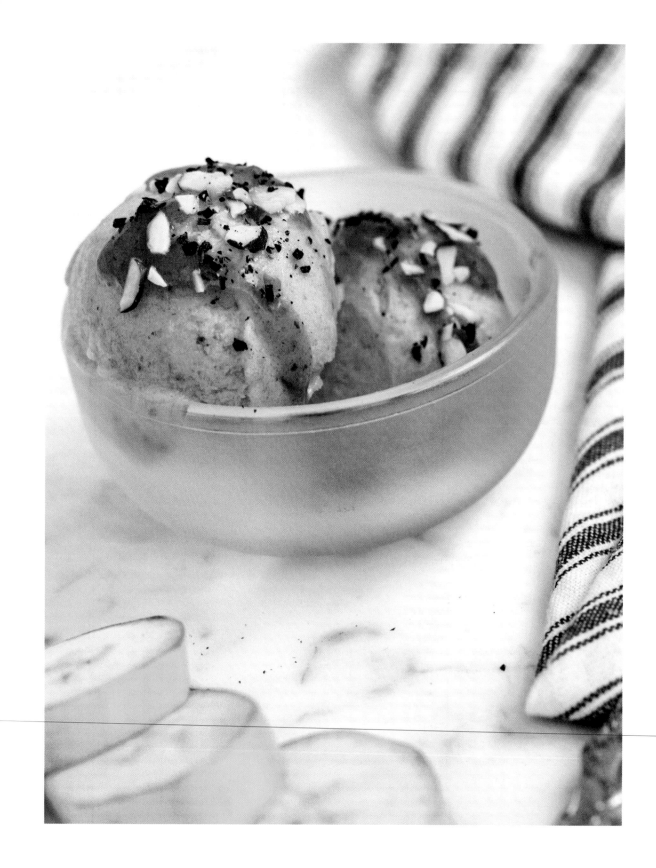

BANANA SOFT SERVE WITH DATE CARAMEL SAUCE

PREP TIME: 10 min

COOK TIME: 0 min

TOTAL TIME: 10 min (does not include freezer time)

MAKES 2 SERVINGS

Move over, ice cream. This deliciously nutritious dessert will leave you convinced it can be good and good for you at the same time.

INGREDIENTS:

3 frozen ripe bananas, sliced into small chunks

Date Caramel Sauce (see recipe on page 328)

PREPARATION:

1. To prepare the frozen bananas, peel and slice the ripe bananas into small chunks. Store in a freezer-safe container in the freezer for 2–3 hours or overnight.

2. Place the frozen banana chunks into a food processor and pulse several times, while occasionally stopping to scrape down the sides. Optional: You can add a splash of almond milk or water to get the blades moving.

3. Keep blending for up to 5 minutes until a creamy consistency is reached. If adding extra ingredients, like nut butters, cocoa powder, chocolate chips, or nuts, this is the time to do it.

4. Serve immediately or return the Banana Soft Serve to the freezer in a freezer-safe container. For a more solid consistency, like ice cream, freeze for an additional hour.

5. When ready to enjoy, serve a scoop and top it with Date Caramel Sauce and/or toppings of choice (like Candied Pecans & Cashews [see recipe on page 237], Chocolate Chip Cookie Dough Bliss Balls [see recipe on page 283], Granola [see recipe on page 60], a dusting of cocoa power, shredded coconut, seeds, nuts, fruit, and chocolate chips.)

PER SERVING WITH 1 TABLESPOON OF SAUCE:
183 calories, 2 grams protein, 47 grams carbohydrates, 1 gram total fat

COCONUT ICE CREAM

PREP TIME: 65 min

COOK TIME: 0 min

TOTAL TIME: 65 min

MAKES 6 SERVINGS

No need for fancy ice-cream equipment to enjoy this rich and delicious dessert. Coconut is a great source of fiber and vitamins A and E, and it helps improve digestion.

INGREDIENTS:

2 13-ounce cans coconut milk

1 cup organic coconut palm sugar or ¾ cup maple syrup

1 teaspoon vanilla extract

shredded coconut, for topping

Date Caramel Sauce (optional) (see recipe on page 328)

PREPARATION:

1. If time permits, refrigerate the cans of coconut milk for a few hours until cold.

2. In a blender, blend all ingredients together until creamy and smooth.

3. Pour the mixture into a freezer-safe bowl or bread pan and store in the freezer for about 30 minutes.

4. Remove the ice cream from the freezer, whisk briefly, and return it to the freezer. Repeat the step one more time until the ice cream is creamy and frozen through.

5. When ready to serve, use an ice-cream scooper to scoop into a bowl. Top the ice cream with shredded coconut and Date Caramel Sauce (optional) and enjoy!

PER SERVING WITHOUT OPTIONAL TOPPINGS:
407 calories, 3 grams protein, 44 grams carbohydrates, 27 grams total fat

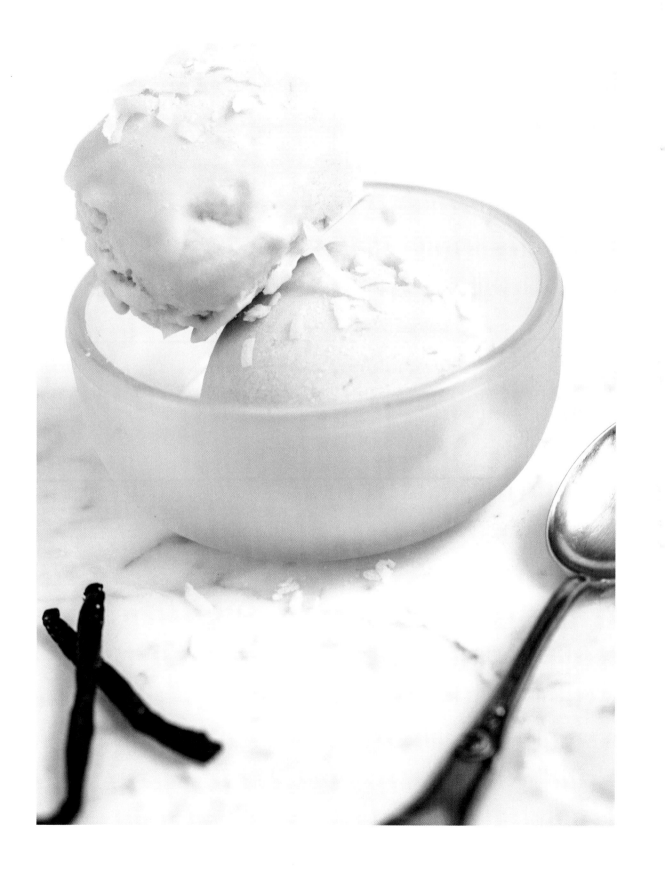

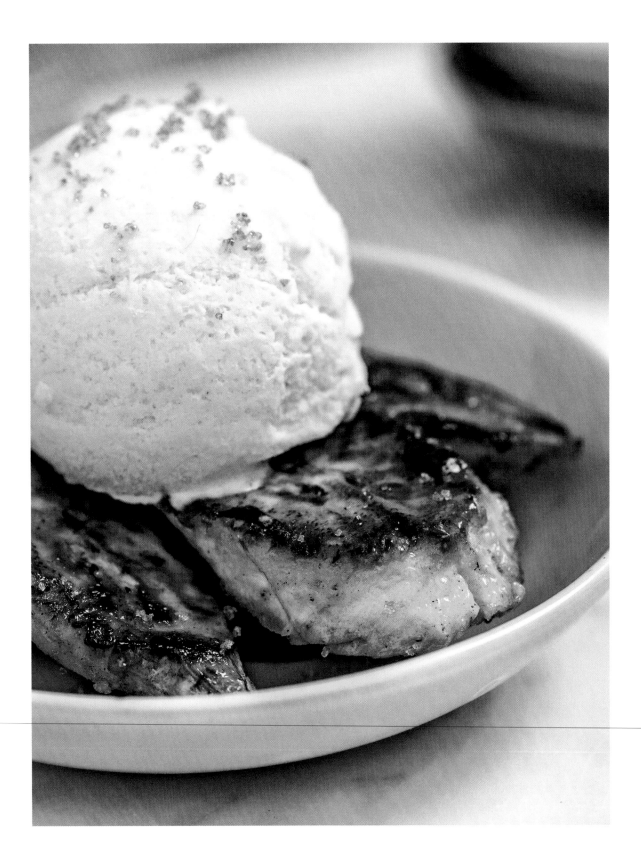

PLÁTANOS MADUROS (SWEET PLANTAINS) À LA MODE

PREP TIME: 5 min

COOK TIME: 8 min

TOTAL TIME: 13 min

MAKES 4 SERVINGS

Plátanos maduros may be new to you, but after this recipe, you may realize love at first bite.

INGREDIENTS:

1 tablespoon coconut oil

2 very ripe plantains, brownish and very tender to the touch

1 tablespoon organic coconut palm sugar or 1 tablespoon maple syrup

pinch of ground cinnamon

Coconut Ice Cream (see recipe on page 300) or Banana Soft Serve (see recipe on page 299)

DIRECTIONS:

1. Heat 1 tablespoon of coconut oil in a large skillet over medium-high heat.

2. Cut off the ends of the plantains and draw a sharp knife along the ridges, lengthwise, making 2–3 slits down the peel from one end to the other.

3. Carefully peel off the skin in sections.

4. Slice each plantain diagonally into ½-inch-thick oval slices. Evenly coat slices with coconut palm sugar or maple syrup and cinnamon.

5. Cook the plantains in the hot skillet for about 4 minutes on each side until soft and caramelized.

6. Serve and top the plantains with a scoop of Coconut Ice Cream or Banana Soft Serve and a sprinkle of coconut palm sugar.

PER SERVING INCLUDING ICE CREAM:
357 calories, 2 grams protein, 54 grams carbohydrates, 17 grams total fat

RAW KEY LIME PIE

▶ **RAW** ▶ **GRAIN-FREE** ▶ **VEGAN**
▶ **NO REFINED SUGAR**

PREP TIME: 30 min

COOK TIME: 0 min

TOTAL TIME: 2 hrs 30 min (includes freezer time but does not include cashew soak time)

MAKES 6 SERVINGS

Key lime pie was my favorite dessert as a kid, so naturally, when I decided to go completely plant-based, I asked my wife to help me get creative so we could find a healthy alternative. She surprised me with the most incredibly delicious, better-than-the-real-thing Raw Key Lime Pie! Enjoy.

INGREDIENTS FOR CRUST:

1 cup organic raw almonds or pecans

1 tablespoon unsweetened shredded coconut

⅛ teaspoon sea salt

6 large organic dates, pitted

1 teaspoon organic unrefined coconut oil

½ teaspoon vanilla extract

1 tablespoon water, add 1 tablespoon at a time if necessary

INGREDIENTS FOR FILLING:

1 cup raw cashews (presoaked in warm water for 1–2 hours)

½ cup vanilla almond milk

½ cup organic lime juice (about 4 limes)

4 tablespoons maple syrup

1 tablespoon organic unrefined coconut oil

½ teaspoon vanilla extract

lime wedges or zest, for garnish

PREPARATION FOR CRUST:

1. In a food processor, process the almonds, shredded coconut, and salt until the consistency is a coarse meal. Then blend in the dates, coconut oil, vanilla extract, and water until well combined.

2. Press the dough evenly and firmly into a 6-cup or 12-cup nonstick cheesecake pan and set in the freezer while preparing the filling.

PREPARATION FOR FILLING:

1. Put all ingredients in a blender and process until smooth.

2. Remove the pan from the freezer and evenly pour the filling on top of the crust.

3. Transfer the pan back to the freezer for about 2 hours or until firm.

4. Remove from the freezer and garnish with lime wedges or lime zest and enjoy!

TIP: Leftovers can be stored in an airtight container in the refrigerator for up to a few days or in the freezer for up to 2 weeks. Thaw for about 20 minutes before serving.

PER SERVING: 374 calories, 9 grams protein, 30 grams carbohydrates, 27 grams total fat

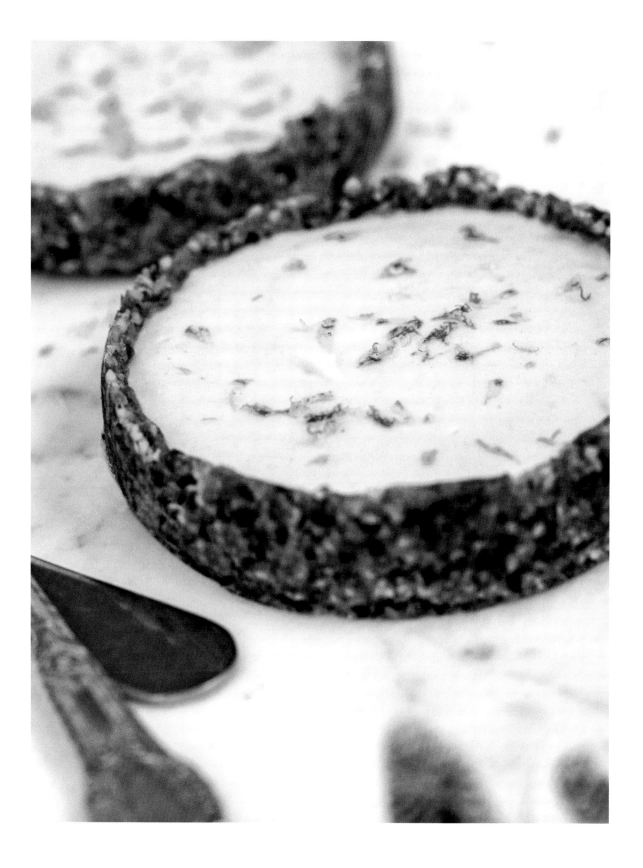

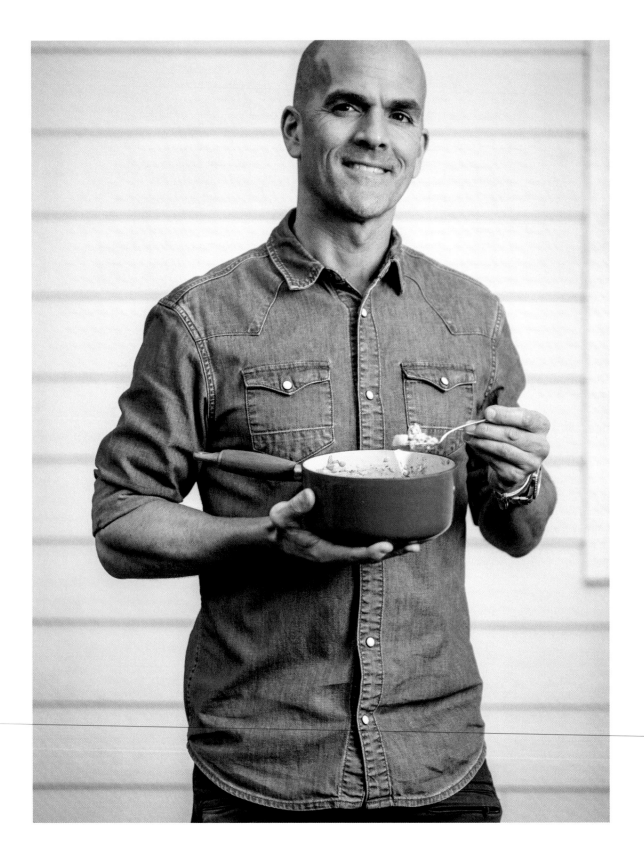

PLANT-BASED BASICS

THE STAPLES OF A plant-based kitchen, like Cashew Cheese and Quinoa, help to make meals a snap. Who doesn't want more time to spend with your family instead of in the kitchen? Instead of relying on standard mixes and sauces to flavor your meals quickly, reach for these healthy, plant-based basics to cut your prep time. These dressings, sauces, and ingredients are the foundation of your plant-based lifestyle.

From Balsamic Vinaigrette Dressing and Creamy Cashew Balsamic Vinaigrette Dressing to Homemade Vanilla Almond Milk and Grandma's Go-To Tomato Sauce, you'll be stocking your pantry with the healthiest versions of your favorite foods. Mozzarella Cheese? Nacho Cheese? That's right. It's all included here for your enjoyment and delight. And having these healthy favorites around will make sticking to your personalized program a snap.

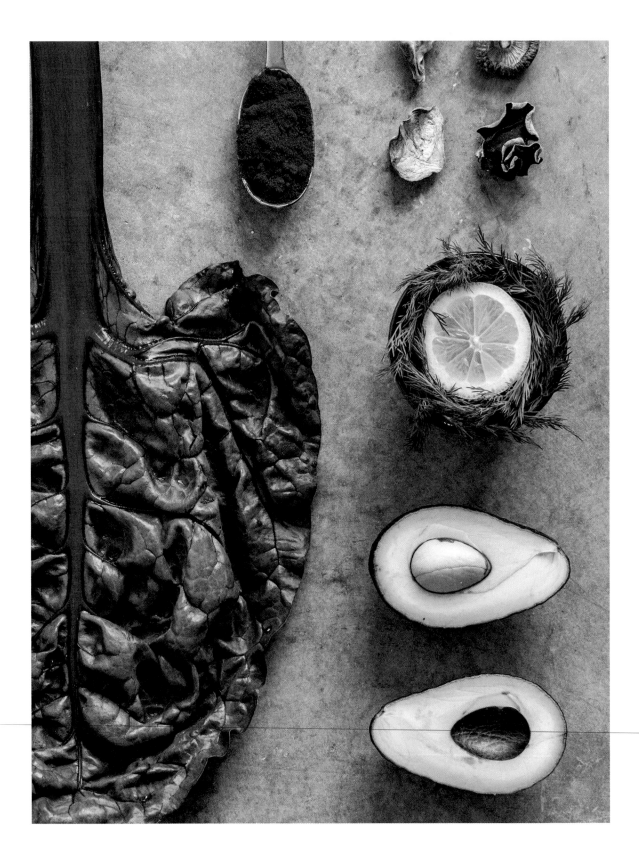

BASIC RECIPES

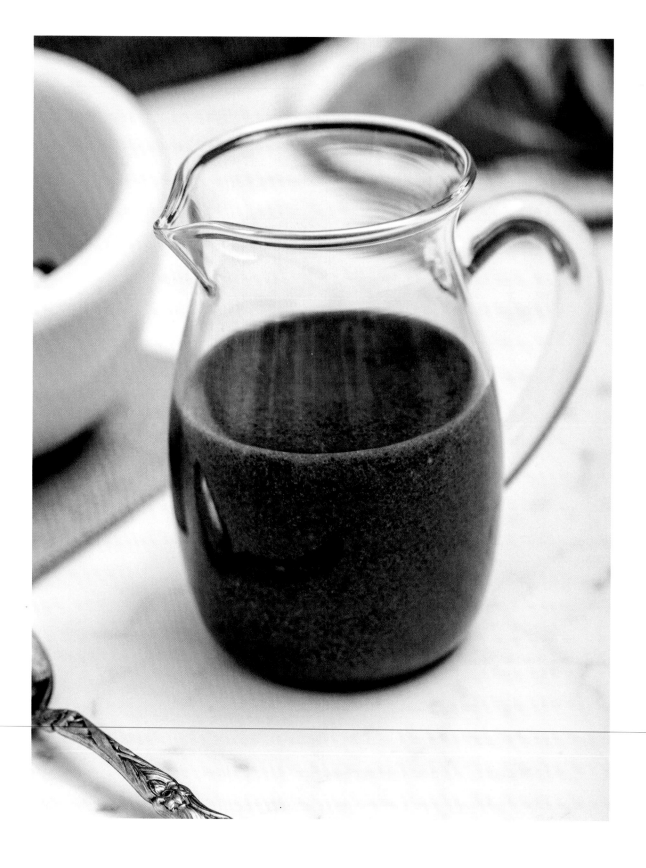

BALSAMIC VINAIGRETTE DRESSING

PREP TIME: 5 min

COOK TIME: 0 min

TOTAL TIME: 5 min

MAKES 8 TABLESPOONS

This is a simple dressing that may soon become a staple in your home. We use it to wet salads and bowls with an added touch of flavor.

INGREDIENTS:

3 tablespoons balsamic vinegar

2 tablespoons extra-virgin olive oil

1 tablespoon water

1 tablespoon lemon juice

1 tablespoon Dijon mustard

1 teaspoon maple syrup

½ teaspoon minced garlic

½ teaspoon sea salt

¼ teaspoon ground black pepper

PREPARATION:

Whisk all ingredients together. Taste and adjust seasoning, as needed.

TIP: This dressing can be made in advance and stored in an airtight glass container in the refrigerator for up to 1 week.

PER 1 TABLESPOON SERVING: 38 calories, 0 grams protein, 2 grams carbohydrates, 3 grams total fat

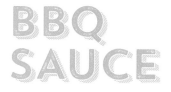

BBQ SAUCE

PREP TIME: 5 min

COOK TIME: 10 min

TOTAL TIME: 15 min

MAKES 2 CUPS

Here's a fresh, homemade BBQ sauce simmered together with simple ingredients. This recipe is delicious with the Black Bean & Quinoa Burger (see recipe on page 153) and the BBQ Meatless Ball Skewers (see recipe on page 189), and it is an essential component in the BBQ Beans (see recipe on page 261).

INGREDIENTS:

1 6-ounce can tomato paste

¾ cup filtered water

4 tablespoons balsamic vinegar

3 tablespoons coconut aminos

2 tablespoons Dijon mustard

1 tablespoon lime juice

¾ teaspoon smoked paprika

¼ teaspoon chili powder

⅛ teaspoon garlic powder

PREPARATION:

1. Combine all ingredients in a saucepan and stir well.

2. Bring to a boil, then reduce to a simmer and cook for about 10 minutes.

TIP: Store the sauce in the refrigerator in an airtight glass container for up to 2 weeks.

PER ¼ CUP SERVING: 34 calories, 1 gram protein, 7 grams carbohydrates, 0 grams total fat

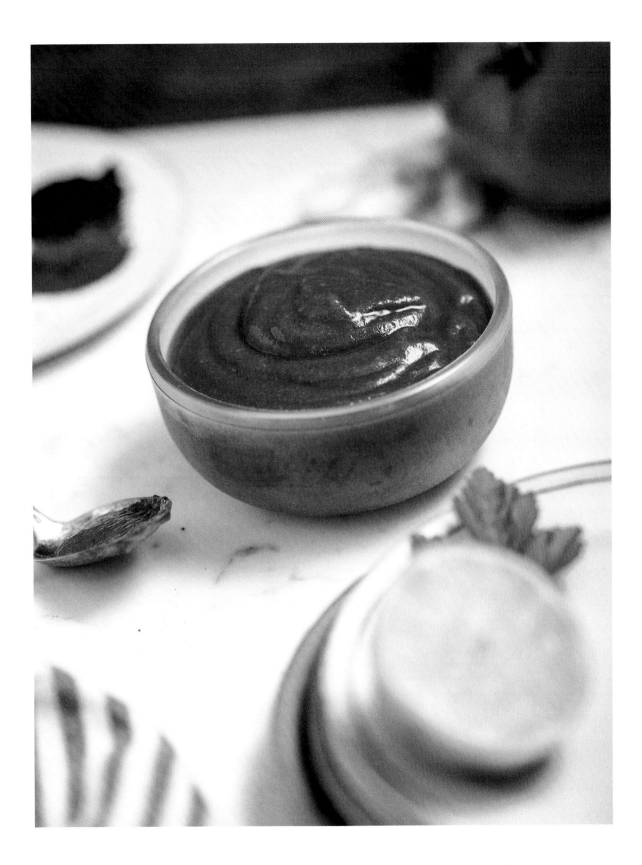

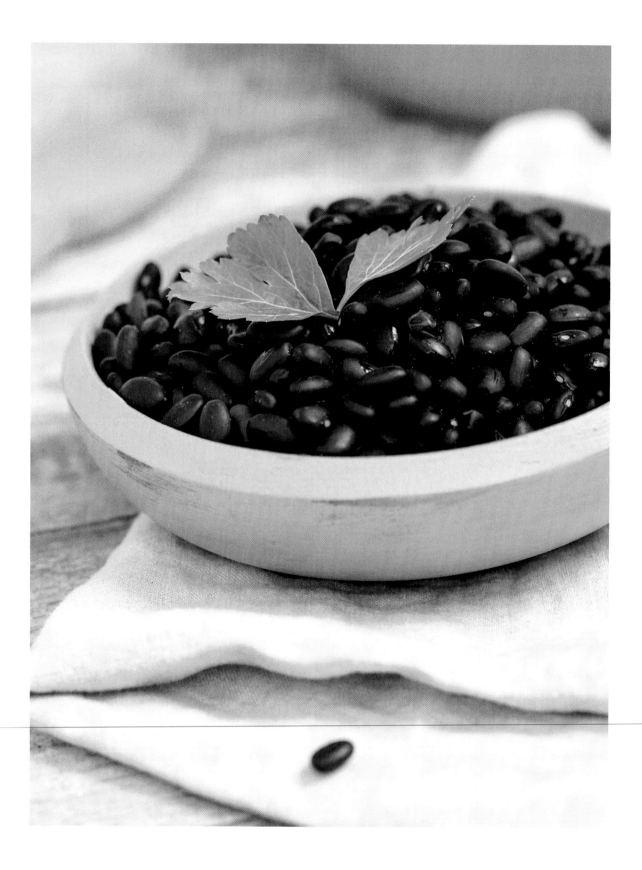

BLACK BEANS

PREP TIME: 5 min
COOK TIME: 90 min
TOTAL TIME: 95 min

MAKES 2½–3 CUPS

We LOVE Beans! Okay, now we got that out there.

Beans can generally take anywhere from 30 minutes to 2 hours to cook, especially black beans. Sometimes adding commonly used acidic ingredients like tomatoes, citrus, vinegar, or lemon juice to the beans before they are fully cooked can prevent the beans from becoming fully tender. This is why it's best to add those ingredients toward the end of the cooking time.

Soaking beans is an important step because it helps reduce the cooking time and also helps break down the indigestible sugars that cause gas. Below are three commonly used methods. The hot-soak method seems to be the most effective.

HOT-SOAK METHOD:

1. Inspect and clean the beans by rinsing in a colander with cold water.

2. Place the beans in a large pot and add 5 cups of water for every cup of beans.

3. Bring to a boil for a few minutes. Remove from heat, cover, and let soak for up to 24 hours.

4. Drain and discard the soaking water.

5. Rinse the beans with fresh water.

TRADITIONAL SOAK METHOD:

1. Inspect and clean the beans by rinsing in a colander with cold water.

2. Soak beans with 3–4 cups of water for every 1 cup of beans.

3. Drain the beans, discard the soaking water, and rinse well with fresh water.

QUICK-SOAK METHOD:

1. Inspect and clean the beans by rinsing in a colander with cold water.

2. Place beans in a large pot with 3–4 cups of water for every 1 cup of beans.

3. Bring to a boil for a few minutes.

4. Remove from heat, cover, and let soak for an hour.

5. Drain the beans and discard the soaking water.

6. Rinse the beans with fresh water.

Recipe continues

TIP: If using the beans as an ingredient for salads, make sure to occasionally stir them while cooking to prevent them from sticking. Also, try to drain the beans immediately after desired tenderness is reached to prevent them from overcooking.

INGREDIENTS:

1 cup black beans, soaked overnight in 3–4 cups of water

2 cups water

sea salt, to taste

PREPARATION:

1. Rinse and drain the beans. In a medium pot, combine the beans with 2 cups of water, and bring to a boil.

2. Reduce the heat to medium-low, cover, and let simmer for 60–90 minutes. Add sea salt to taste, 45 minutes through the cooking time.

3. When the desired consistency is reached, remove the beans from the heat and enjoy!

PER ¾ CUP COOKED SERVING: 165 calories, 10 grams protein, 30 grams carbohydrates, 1 gram total fat

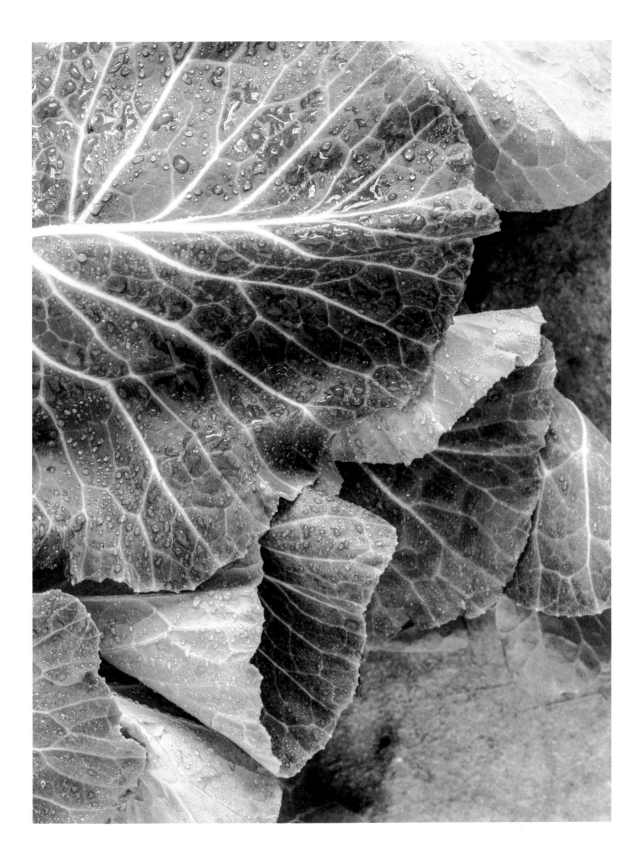

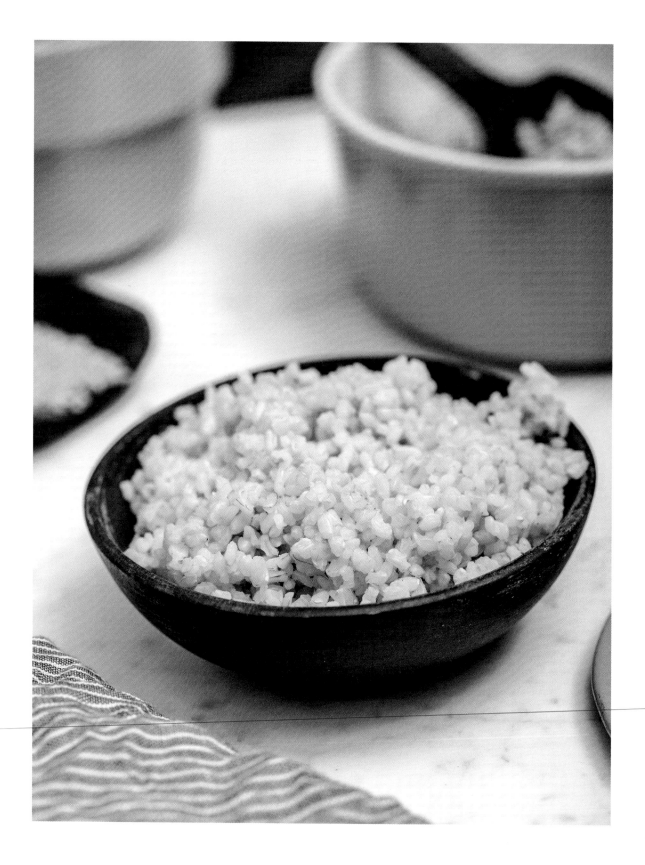

SHORT-GRAIN BROWN RICE

PREP TIME: 5 min

COOK TIME: 55 min

TOTAL TIME: 60 min

MAKES 3 CUPS

This rice is an excellent source of whole grains. It has a sticky texture once cooked, and this can come in handy when making different recipes.

INGREDIENTS:

1 cup short-grain brown rice

2 cups water

½ teaspoon sea salt

PREPARATION:

1. In a medium pot, combine the rice, water, and salt and bring to a boil.

2. Stir once, reduce the heat to low, cover, and let simmer for about 55 minutes. If the rice seems too dry, then add up to ¼ of a cup of water and cook a little longer.

3. Remove from the heat and keep the rice covered until ready to enjoy.

4. Fluff with a fork and serve!

PER ¾ CUP COOKED SERVING: 164 calories, 3 grams protein, 34 grams carbohydrates, 1 gram total fat

CASHEW CHEESE

PREP TIME: 10 min

COOK TIME: 0 min

TOTAL TIME: 10 min

MAKES 1½ CUPS

This "cheese" is very versatile and convenient to have in the refrigerator on hand. It can be used as cheese and for dressings, dips, sauces, and other preparations. Once you notice how many times this Cashew Cheese is used in our recipes, you'll always want to have it on hand.

For a simple cheddar cheese, just add turmeric. You can use this variation for Mac 'n' Cheese by adding a little pasta water. For Alfredo sauce, add about ½ cup pasta water. To make a salad dressing, whisk in Dijon mustard, water, and the seasonings of your choice. Or simply drizzle this cheese over soups and watch it work its magic.

INGREDIENTS:

1 cup raw cashews, presoaked in water overnight

¼ cup water

3 tablespoons nutritional yeast

1 tablespoon lime juice

1 tablespoon apple cider vinegar

½ teaspoon sea salt

PREPARATION:

Drain and rinse the cashews, then toss them into the blender (or food processor) with the rest of the ingredients. Blend until smooth. If pressed for time, soak cashews in warm water for about 30 minutes, then drain and rinse.

TIP: Store Cashew Cheese in an airtight glass container in the refrigerator for up to a week. It will harden slightly when chilled.

PER ¼ CUP SERVING: 165 calories, 6 grams protein, 9 grams carbohydrates, 12 grams total fat

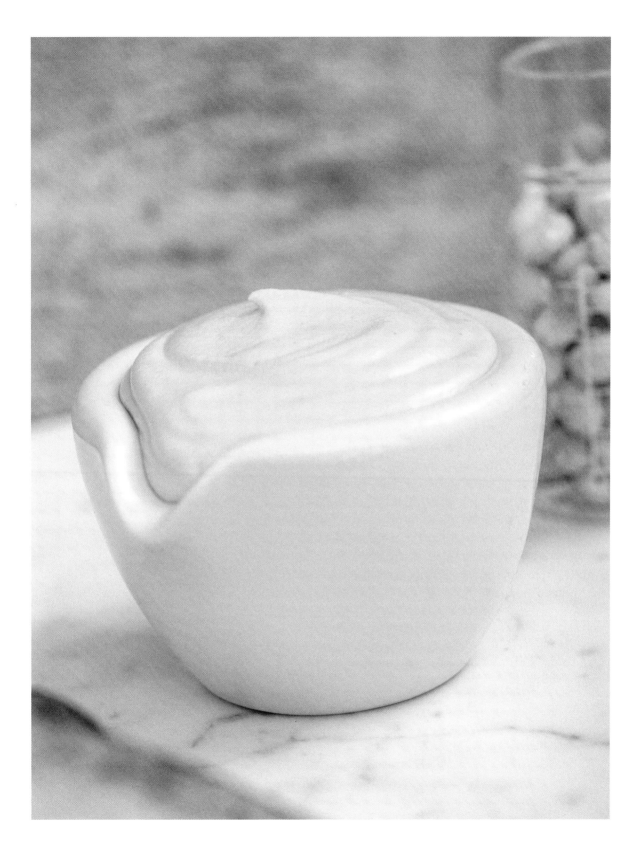

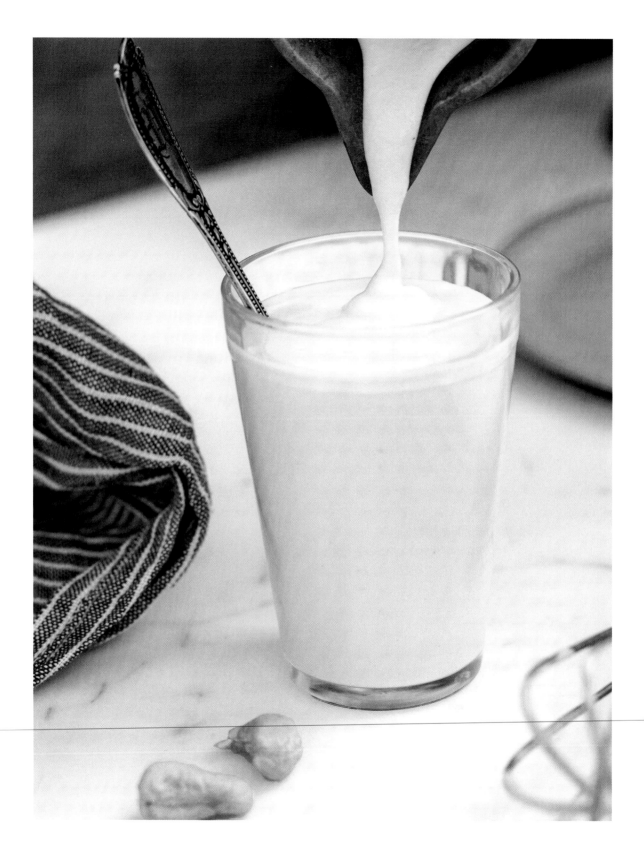

CASHEW CREAM SAUCE/ DRESSING

PREP TIME: 5 min

COOK TIME: 0 min

TOTAL TIME: 5 min (does not include cashew soak time)

MAKES 1 CUP

This is a slightly modified version of our Cashew Cheese with a multitude of uses. The thinner consistency allows for use as a light dressing over salads and bowls.

INGREDIENTS:

½ cup raw cashews, presoaked in water overnight

½ cup water

1 tablespoon nutritional yeast

1 tablespoon lime juice

½ teaspoon sea salt or to taste

PREPARATION:

Drain and rinse the cashews, then toss them into a blender or food processor with the rest of the ingredients. Blend until smooth. If pressed for time, soak the cashews in warm water for about 30 minutes, then drain and rinse.

TIP: Leftovers can be stored in an airtight glass container in the refrigerator for up to 1 week. This recipe is used in the Tomato Basil Cream Pasta (see recipe on page 223) and the Penne Pasta with Spinach Cream Sauce (see recipe on page 220).

PER ¼ CUP SERVING: 122 calories, 4 grams protein, 7 grams carbohydrates, 9 grams total fat

COCONUT WHIPPED CREAM

PREP TIME: 10 min

COOK TIME: 0 min

TOTAL TIME: 10 min

MAKES 8 SERVINGS

Coconut Whipped Cream adds a touch of richness to any dish. Enjoy this over fruit, pancakes, muffins, cakes, other desserts, and even hot cocoa.

INGREDIENTS:

1 can chilled full-fat coconut milk

2 tablespoons maple syrup or to taste

1 teaspoon vanilla extract

PREPARATION:

1. Refrigerate coconut milk overnight. This helps firm up the cream.

2. When ready to use, remove the can from the refrigerator and flip it upside down.

3. Open the can and pour the liquid into a container for later use (perfect for smoothies).

4. Scoop out the solid coconut cream from the can into a mixing bowl and beat using an electric hand mixer or stand mixer.

5. Add the maple syrup and vanilla extract and whip again until the cream is smooth and fluffy.

TIP: Store in an airtight container or mason jar in the refrigerator for about 1 week. Whisk gently when ready to use again. For a Chocolate Coconut Whipped Cream, add 4 tablespoons cocoa powder.

PER SERVING: 101 calories, 1 gram protein, 5 grams carbohydrates, 10 grams total fat

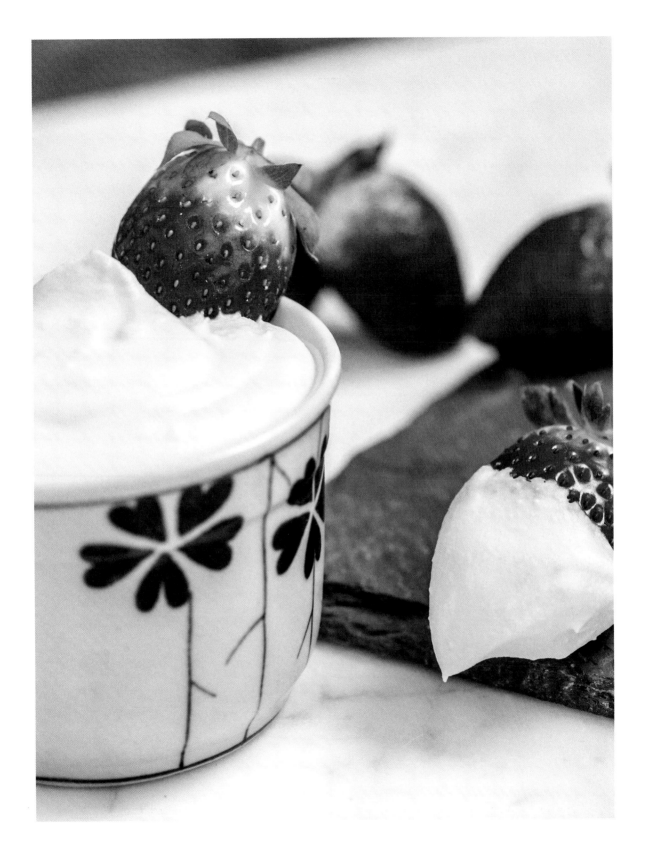

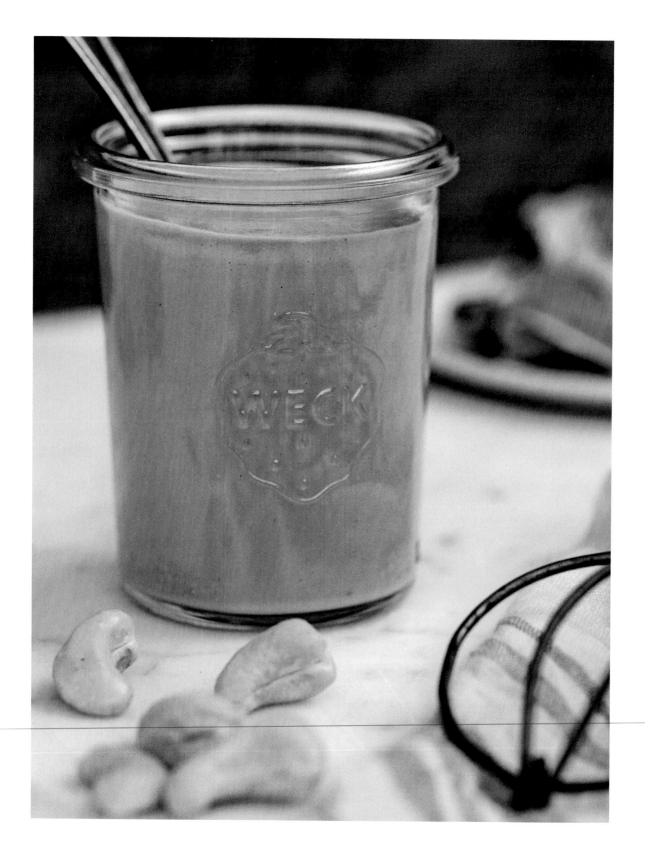

CREAMY CASHEW BALSAMIC VINAIGRETTE DRESSING

PREP TIME: 5 min

COOK TIME: 0 min

TOTAL TIME: 5 min

MAKES 1 CUP

I love this dressing over my quinoa bowls and salads.

INGREDIENTS:

½ cup raw cashews, presoaked in water overnight

½ cup water

4 tablespoons balsamic vinegar

1 tablespoon Dijon mustard

½ teaspoon sea salt or to taste

PREPARATION:

Drain and rinse the cashews, then toss them in a blender or food processor with the rest of the ingredients. Blend until smooth. If pressed for time, soak the cashews in warm water for about 30 minutes, then drain and rinse.

TIP: Leftovers can be stored in an airtight glass container in the refrigerator for up to 1 week.

PER 1 TABLESPOON SERVING: 34 calories, 1 gram protein, 2 grams carbohydrates, 2 grams total fat

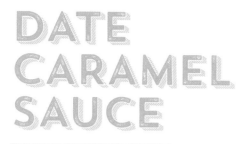

DATE CARAMEL SAUCE

PREP TIME: 35 min

COOK TIME: 0 min

TOTAL TIME: 35 min

MAKES ½ CUP

Dates are an excellent source of fiber, potassium, and magnesium, which make this a functional topping you'll love over pancakes, desserts, muffins, and bread.

INGREDIENTS:

8 Medjool dates, pitted and presoaked in warm water for 30 min.

½ cup sweetened vanilla almond milk, adding more if necessary

PREPARATION:

1. Drain the dates and transfer to a high-speed blender or food processor and blend together with the almond milk until smooth and creamy. Add more almond milk, one tablespoon at a time, if you prefer a thinner consistency.

2. Serve the sauce immediately.

TIP: Leftovers can be stored in an airtight container in the refrigerator for up to 3 days.

PER 1 TABLESPOON SERVING: 26 calories, 0 grams protein, 6 grams carbohydrates, 0 grams total fat

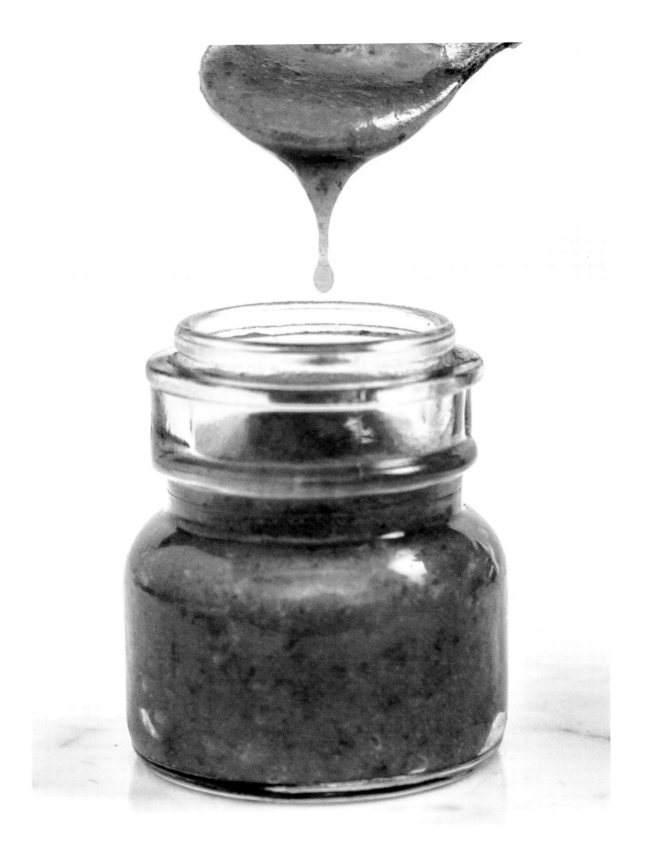

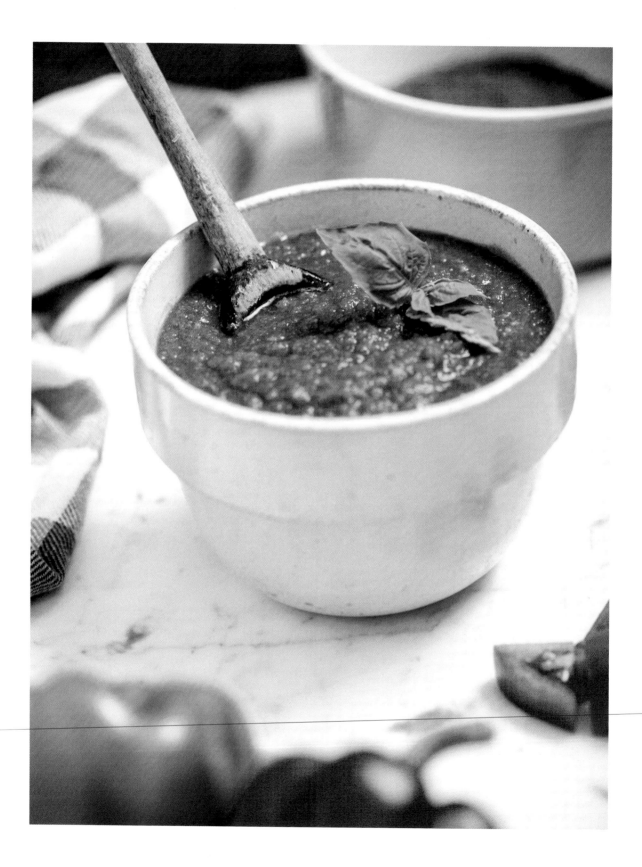

GRANDMA'S GO-TO TOMATO SAUCE

PREP TIME: 10 min

COOK TIME: 30 min

TOTAL TIME: 40 min

MAKES ABOUT 6 CUPS

There are so many uses for this tomato sauce, we could give it a chapter. Tomatoes are rich in B vitamins, vitamins C and K, biotin, potassium, fiber, manganese, and antioxidants, which make it a powerhouse ingredient on its own. Add to that the bounty of other vegetables found in this sauce, and you have yourself a nutritional superpower.

INGREDIENTS:

2 pounds ripe tomatoes, washed, cored, and chopped, or 4–5 large tomatoes

1 large carrot, washed and chopped (about ½ cup)

1 small red pepper, washed, cored, seeded, and chopped

1 green pepper, washed, cored, seeded, and chopped

1 small onion, chopped

1 clove garlic (1 teaspoon minced)

4 fresh basil leaves or 1 teaspoon dried basil flakes

½ to 1 teaspoon sea salt, or to taste

dash cayenne pepper

PREPARATION:

1. Add all ingredients into a blender and, working in batches, blend until smooth.

2. Pour the sauce into a large pot and cook at medium-low heat, stirring often, for 25–30 minutes, skimming off any foam that may rise to the top. The sauce will darken as it cooks. Taste and adjust seasoning, if necessary.

TIP: Store leftover sauce in an airtight container in the fridge for up to 5 days or in the freezer for a few months. It is best if stored in portion-size containers to prolong freshness. This way you touch only the sauce you are using each time.

PER ½ CUP SERVING: 22 calories, 1 gram protein, 5 grams carbohydrates, 0 grams total fat

HOMEMADE VANILLA ALMOND MILK

PREP TIME: 15 min

COOK TIME: 0 min

TOTAL TIME: 15 min

MAKES 3 CUPS

Commercial nut milks/drinks are usually full of sugar and come with a long list of ingredients. This almond milk is simple and easy to make without the excess sugar or extra ingredients.

INGREDIENTS:

1 cup raw almonds

3 cups water

1 tablespoon maple syrup

1 teaspoon vanilla extract

PREPARATION:

1. Presoak the raw almonds in 2 cups of water overnight.

2. Rinse the almonds and blend with 3 cups of water until smooth and creamy.

3. Strain the almond mixture into a large bowl through a nut milk bag, sprouting bag, or cheesecloth. (Reserve the almond pulp to make Almond Pulp Cookies [see recipe on page 292].)

4. Pour the almond milk back into the blender and add the maple syrup and vanilla. Blend until well combined.

TIP: Store in a glass jar or pitcher in the refrigerator for up to 4 days. Stir well when ready to use.

PER 1 CUP SERVING: 80 calories, 12 grams protein, 2 grams carbohydrates, 3 grams total fat

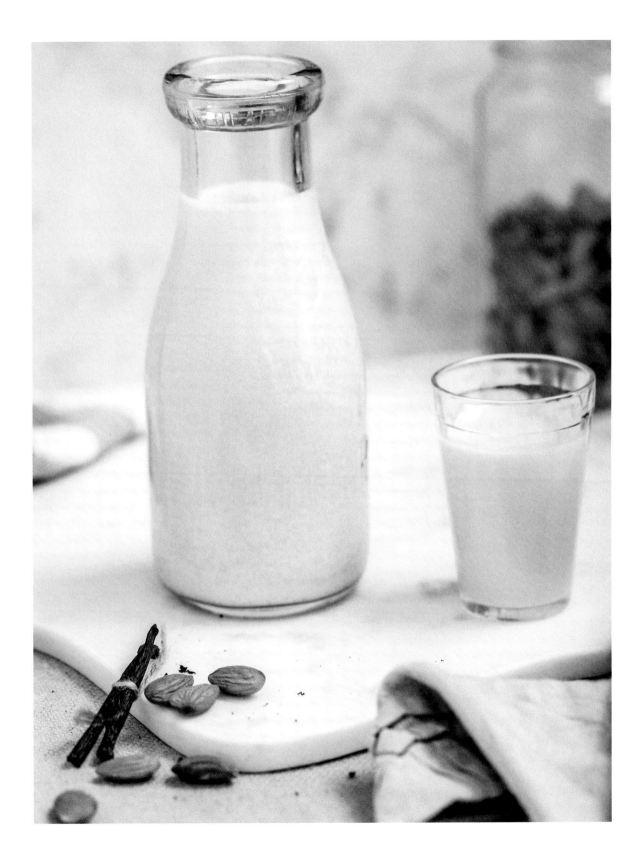

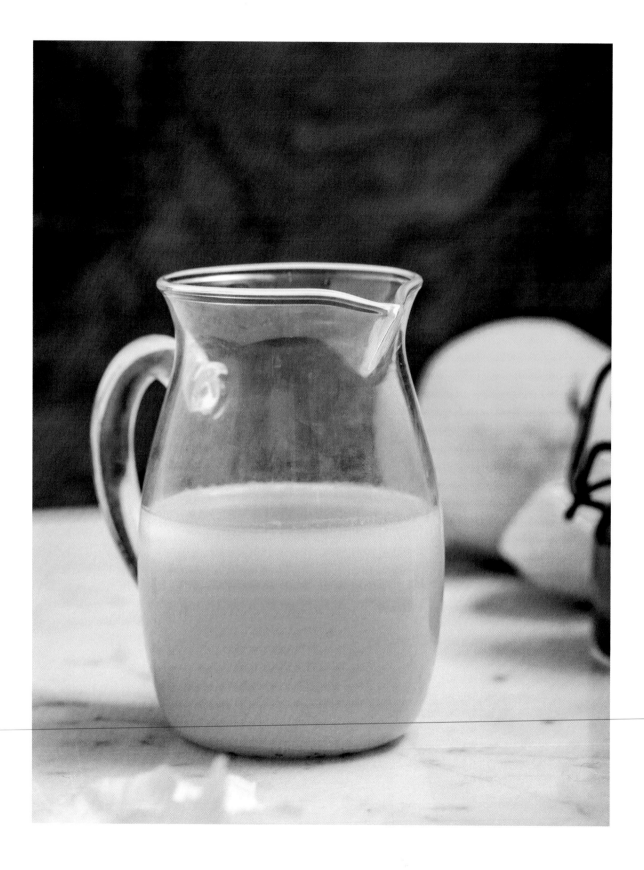

LEMON DIJON VINAIGRETTE DRESSING

PREP TIME: 5 min

COOK TIME: 0 min

TOTAL TIME: 5 min

MAKES ½ CUP

This lemon vinaigrette is a great touch of flavor for light salads.

INGREDIENTS:

4 tablespoons lemon juice

2 tablespoons extra-virgin olive oil

1 tablespoon Dijon mustard

1 tablespoon water

½ teaspoon garlic, minced

½ teaspoon sea salt

¼ teaspoon ground black pepper

PREPARATION:

In a bowl, whisk together all ingredients. Taste and adjust seasoning, as needed.

TIP: The dressing can be made in advance and stored in an airtight glass container in the refrigerator for up to 1 week.

PER 1 TABLESPON SERVING: 33 calories, 0 grams protein, 1 gram carbohydrate, 3 grams total fat

MOZZARELLA CHEESE

PREP TIME: 5 min

COOK TIME: 5 min

TOTAL TIME: 10 min

MAKES 1 CUP

This recipe is easy to make and very versatile. Use it when making pizza, dips, grilled cheese sandwiches—you name it. Make it fresh or have it premade in the refrigerator until you're ready to use it. If using the recipe for a dip, reheat it in a saucepan over medium-high heat, stirring often and making sure it doesn't burn. If the consistency is too thick, add water, 1 tablespoon at a time.

INGREDIENTS:

½ cup raw cashews, presoaked in water overnight

1 cup water

1 tablespoon tapioca flour

1 teaspoon lemon juice

1 teaspoon apple cider vinegar

½ teaspoon sea salt

PREPARATION:

1. Drain and rinse the cashews, then toss them into a blender or food processor with the rest of the ingredients. Blend until smooth. If pressed for time, soak the cashews in warm water for about 30 minutes, then drain and rinse.

2. In a saucepan, cook the cheese for about 5 minutes, stirring often over medium-high heat.

3. Reduce the heat and keep stirring to prevent the cheese from clumping and burning.

4. Once consistency has thickened and the mixture looks like melted cheese, remove from the heat and let cool.

TIP: Leftovers can be stored in an airtight container in the fridge for up to 5 days.

PER ¼ CUP SERVING: 127 calories, 4 grams protein, 9 grams carbohydrates, 9 grams total fat

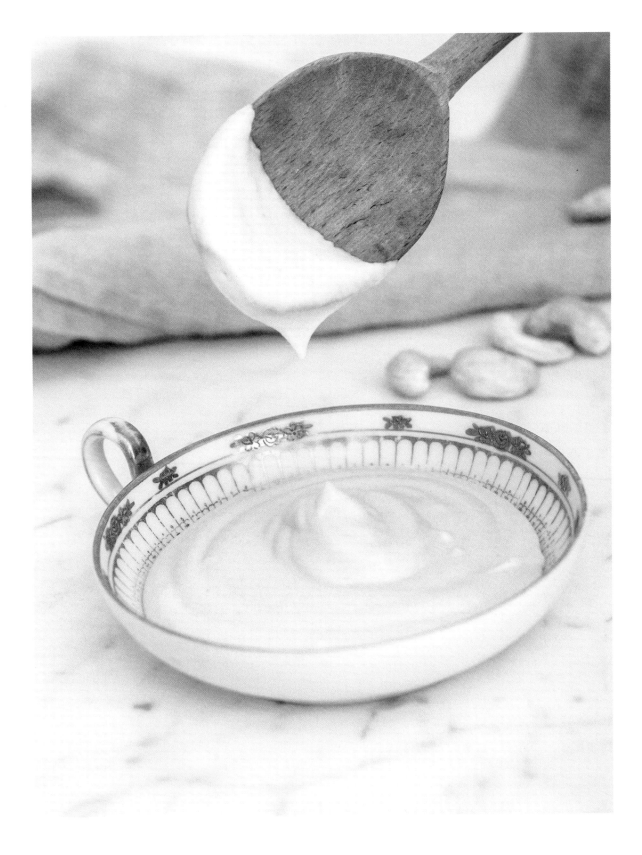

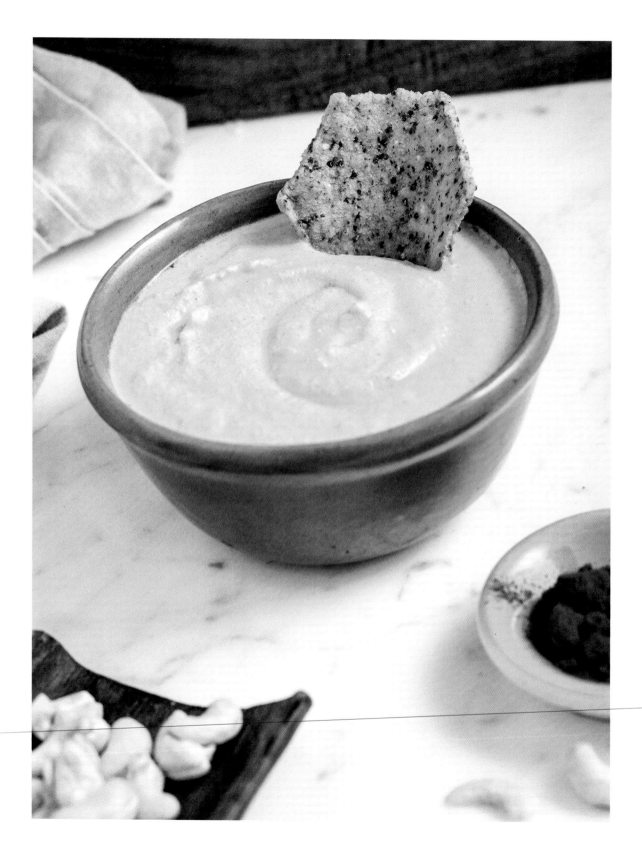

NACHO CHEESE

PREP TIME: 10 min

COOK TIME: 0 min

TOTAL TIME: 10 min

MAKES 2 CUPS

This cheese can be used in many recipes or simply enjoyed as a dip with chips. Make it fresh or make it ahead of time and store it in the refrigerator. When ready to use, reheat the cheese in a saucepan over medium-high heat, stirring often and making sure it doesn't burn. If the consistency is too thick, add water, 1 tablespoon at a time.

INGREDIENTS:

1½ cups Cashew Cheese (see recipe on page 320)

1 medium tomato, peeled, seeded, and roughly chopped

½ cup onion, chopped

½ teaspoon turmeric

½ teaspoon smoked paprika

¼ teaspoon cayenne pepper

PREPARATION:

Add all ingredients to a blender or food processor and blend until smooth.

TIP: Store cheese in an airtight glass container in the refrigerator for up to 1 week. It will harden slightly when chilled.

PER 1 TABLESPOON SERVING: 33 calories, 1 gram protein, 2 grams carbohydrates, 2 grams total fat

PARMESAN CHEESE

PREP TIME: 5 min

COOK TIME: 0 min

TOTAL TIME: 5 min

MAKES 1 CUP

This Parmesan is extremely versatile and great over pastas, salads, avocados, and walnut crumble.

INGREDIENTS:

1 cup raw cashews or blanched almonds

2 tablespoons nutritional yeast

½ teaspoon sea salt

PREPARATION:

Combine all ingredients in a food processor and pulse until a fine meal is formed. Be careful not to overprocess.

TIP: Store this cheese in an airtight container in the refrigerator for up to a few weeks or in the freezer for up to 6 months.

PER 1 TABLESPOON SERVING: 61 calories, 2 grams protein, 3 grams carbohydrates, 5 grams total fat

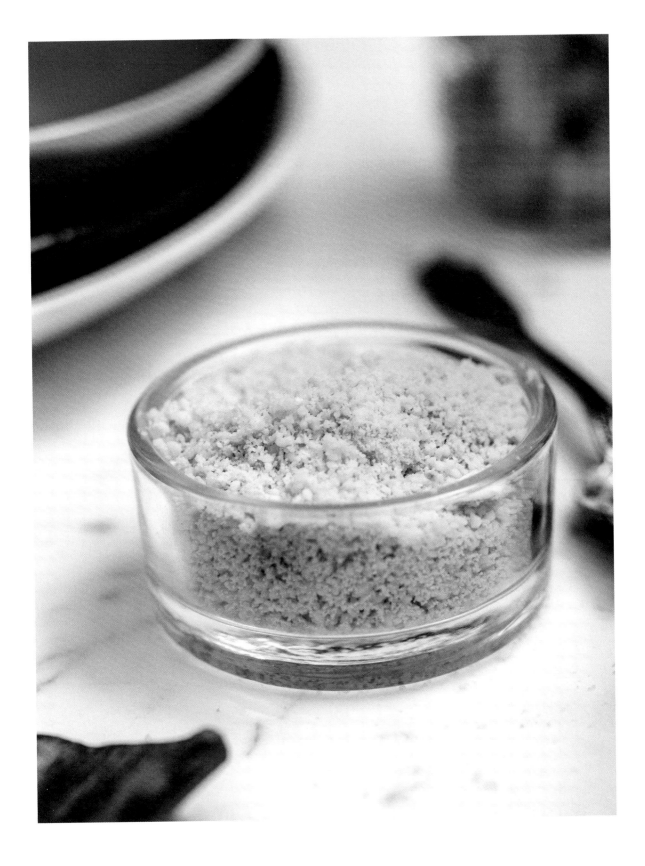

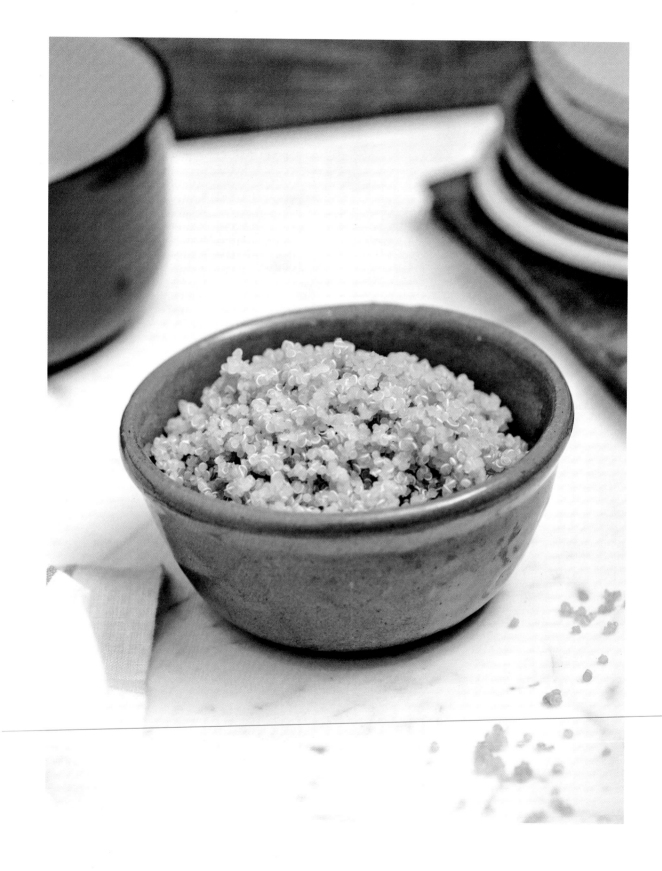

QUINOA

PREP TIME: 5 min
COOK TIME: 25 min
TOTAL TIME: 30 min

MAKES 3 CUPS

Quinoa, which is often called a grain, is actually a gluten-free super seed that comes from the Chenopodium or goosefoot plant. It's easily digestible and provides about 8 grams of protein and 5 grams of fiber per cooked cup. Quinoa is a complete protein that offers all nine essential amino acids. It is packed with vitamins and minerals like the B vitamin thiamin (13 percent), riboflavin (12 percent), folate (19 percent), and vitamin B_6 (11 percent). It's also a rich source of iron (15 percent), phosphorus (28 percent), magnesium (30 percent), manganese (58 percent), copper (18 percent), and zinc (13 percent), as well as potassium (9 percent), vitamin E (6 percent), and the B vitamin niacin (4 percent). And for this, quinoa is a nutritional powerhouse staple in our home!

INGREDIENTS:

1 cup quinoa, uncooked and rinsed

2 cups water

½ teaspoon sea salt

PREPARATION:

1. In a medium saucepan, combine the quinoa, water, and salt and bring to a boil.

2. Reduce the heat to medium-low, cover, and simmer for about 25–30 minutes.

3. Fluff with a fork, remove from the heat, and cover until ready to enjoy!

PER ½ CUP COOKED SERVING: 104 calories, 4 grams protein, 18 grams carbohydrates, 2 grams total fat

TAHINI DRESSING

PREP TIME: 5 min

COOK TIME: 0 min

TOTAL TIME: 5 min

MAKES ½ CUP

This is by far my favorite dressing and the one I most often use. It's simple, delicious, and loaded with manganese, calcium, magnesium, fiber, selenium, zinc, and iron.

INGREDIENTS:

4 tablespoons tahini

4 tablespoons lemon juice

1 tablespoon distilled vinegar

sea salt, to taste

PREPARATION:

In a bowl, stir together all ingredients until creamy and smooth.

TIP: The dressing can be made in advance and stored in an airtight glass container in the refrigerator for up to 1 week.

PER 1 TABLESPOON SERVING: 45 calories, 1 gram protein, 2 grams carbohydrates, 4 grams total fat

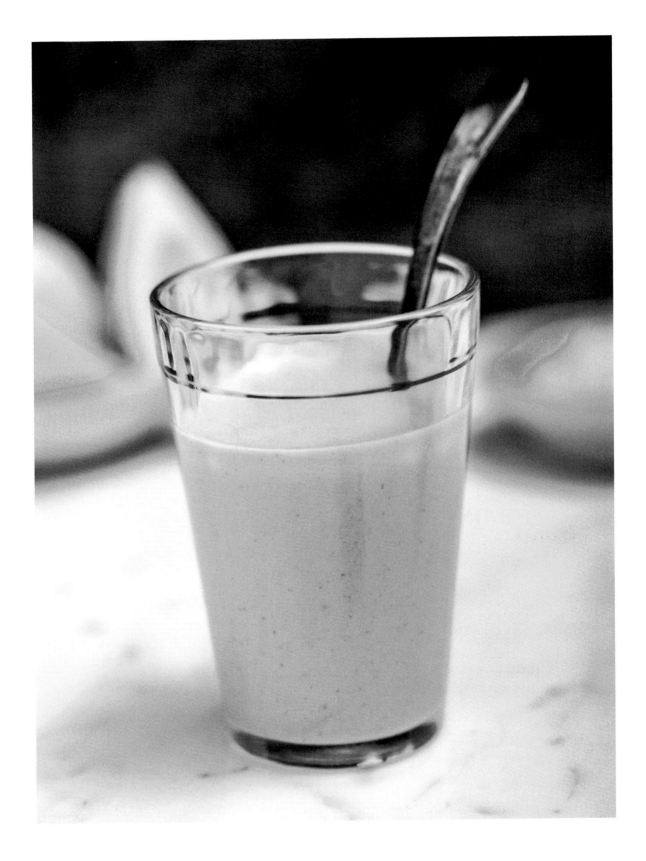

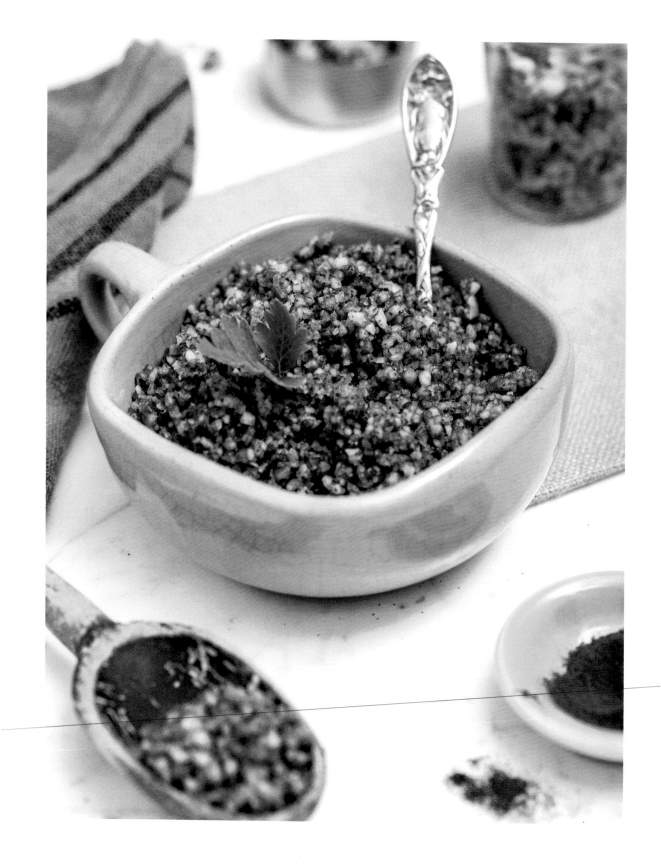

WALNUT MEAT

PREP TIME: 10 min
COOK TIME: 0 min
TOTAL TIME: 10 min

MAKES 1 CUP

This recipe is so versatile and a great addition to many of our meals. In our home, we make it weekly and store it in a mason jar to have on hand for many of our recipes, including Walnut Chili (see recipe on page 227), Walnut Bean Burgers (see recipe on page 159), and Loaded Baked Potato (see recipe on page 183). Walnuts are a great source of heart-healthy omega-3 fatty acids.

INGREDIENTS:

1 cup raw walnuts, roughly chopped

1 tablespoon balsamic vinegar

½ tablespoon coconut aminos

¾ tablespoon ground cumin

½ tablespoon ground coriander

dash smoked paprika

dash garlic powder

dash ground black pepper

dash sea salt

PREPARATION:

Combine all ingredients in a food processor and pulse several times until crumbly. Do not overblend.

TIP: Store in an airtight container in the refrigerator until ready to use. For optimum flavor, best if used within 4–5 days.

PER 1 TABLESPOON SERVING: 176 calories, 4 grams protein, 5 grams carbohydrates, 17 grams total fat

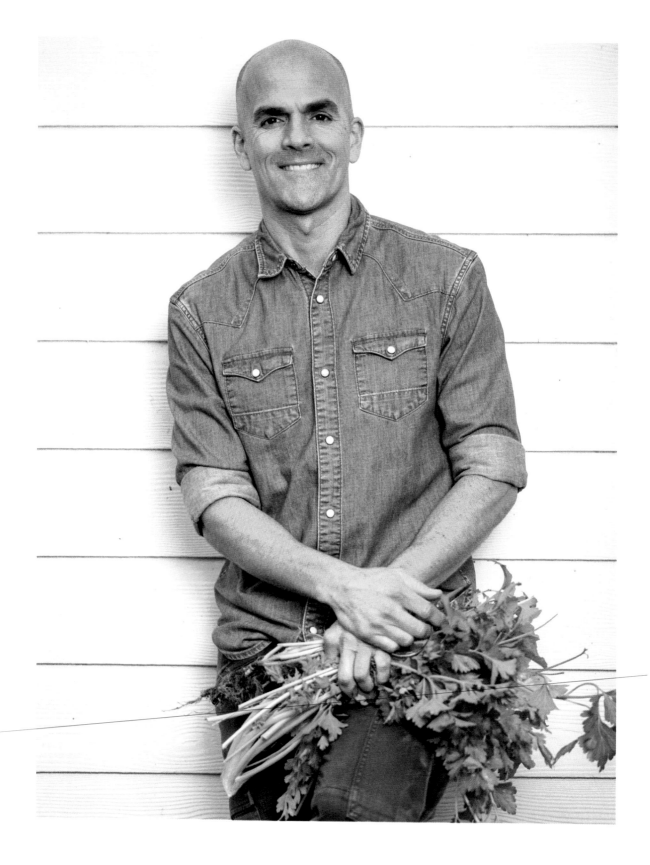

RESTAURANT GUIDE

THERE ARE MANY MISCONCEPTIONS about eating plant-based, one of them being "you can't eat out." When you are beginning any new healthy lifestyle, you're faced with many of the unhealthy foods you used to love. However, the key is understanding that choosing unhealthy foods is a habit. After you commit to the 22-Day Program, you will develop new habits that will allow you to go to almost all of your favorite restaurants, just with different order preferences.

Yes, plant-based eaters go to restaurants! You will not miss out or feel deprived if you initially put in a little extra effort to set yourself up for success. Most restaurants have vegetable-based pasta dishes, hearty salads, and veggie plates on the menu, and some even have an entire section for vegetarian dishes that are easy enough to make vegan.

My dear friend Raymond, whom I previously wrote about losing seventy pounds, has kept the weight off for more than two years! What's most interesting is that he used to eat out ten to twelve meals a week in restaurants—almost every meal—and never even had a plant-based side dish. Today, he is still a huge foodie, but now prefers plant-based foods. He goes out almost as much and to most of the same restaurants. Granted, he now seeks out new chefs and restaurants because of his newfound love of plant-based foods. However, he still defers to friends, family, and clients on restaurants—fully confident that he will always find great food options or rely on the chef for a special dish. He is a true testament that your social life doesn't end with a plant-based diet. In fact, you'll love going out even more and will usually be just as happy when you're ordering as when you're done with your meal. Before 22 days, he would be excited when he ordered, but then overeat and hate himself after. Sometimes, he even would even avoid plans because he knew he would abuse himself with food. Now he is liberated. Eating out no longer means eating terribly. He now enjoys life with fewer restrictions and food with more pleasure than ever.

Just because you can eat almost everywhere doesn't mean you should avoid amazing plant-focused restaurants. Introduce your friends to all of the delicious flavors you are enjoying and share the health benefits. There are more and more of them opening throughout the country and the world, featuring many healthy and indulgent options. Vegans AND nonvegans love them!

And remember: When you're out with family and friends, you're primarily there for the people, so relax and have a great time socializing instead of obsessing over food.

Here are some simple things you can do to find healthy options that still fit your new eating plan.

- If you're in between a few places, Google the menus.
- If you're specifically looking for vegan restaurants, there are several apps you can download, such as HappyCow (my favorite).
- Don't go starving! Ordering with hungry eyes can lead to overeating, so have a small, healthy snack, such as a handful of almonds, before you go.
- Look for healthful, clean food. Things that are made of vegetables, as close to the earth as possible: fresh salads, vegetable side dishes that are cooked or steamed lightly, vegetable soups, brown rice.
- Order salad dressing on the side and add it to taste, or get oil and vinegar and add it yourself.
- Don't be afraid to ask questions and to request substitutions or alternative methods of preparing a dish. Be polite, of course, and more often than not, a restaurant can accommodate your request. Keep in mind that restaurants and chefs won't know what people want unless we request it.
- Order fresh fruit for dessert.

These are some of my go-to options when we eat out. No matter where you go, there are always possibilities if you get creative and advocate for your needs. Enjoy!

BREAKFAST

- Cereals: Most cereals are loaded with sugar, so we tend to stay away from them and instead lean toward healthier options like muesli topped with berries and enjoyed with almond or another nut-based milk. (Rice milk is another great alternative if you're allergic to nuts.)

- Fruit salad
- Oatmeal, with some berries
- Veggie breakfast wrap with beans and avocado
- Avocado toast
- Acai bowls

AMERICAN

- Veggie burger, with or without bread; ask for chopped tomatoes and avocados on top
- Grilled veggies and brown rice or quinoa
- Veggie platter, or if they don't have this on the menu, try building your own from the sides
- Salads, dressing on the side, and don't forget to say, "Hold the cheese!"
- Soups, particularly red lentil, split pea, and nondairy butternut squash

MEXICAN

- Start with guacamole, replacing chips with jicama, carrots, celery, or other crudités.
- Soups like black bean soup or gazpacho
- Veggie fajitas with salsa

ITALIAN

- Start with lightly sautéed artichokes with garlic or minestrone soup.
- Thin-crust pizza becomes bruschetta with veggie toppings like tomato with garlic, spinach or broccoli rabe, or mushrooms and a dash of fresh ground pepper. Hold the cheese!
- Pasta primavera with garlic and a light hint of olive oil or a marinara sauce (without dairy)

ASIAN

- Start with sushi vegetable rolls such as cucumber and avocado, mango and asparagus, and sweet potato; seaweed salad; or lemongrass or coconut soup.
- Vegetable pad thai, vegetable curries, and vegetable rice dishes
- Steamed or lightly sautéed veggies with brown rice
- Make sure to ask for no egg, no fish sauce (in everything), and that the curry paste used is vegan.

GREEK

- Start with appetizers like hummus, usually served with pitas but try with veggie crudités too; tahini, olives, pita bread, stuffed grape leaves (the veggie kind).
- Greek salad
- Make your own vegetable plate of sides like roasted eggplant, grilled veggies, and pan-fried potatoes.
- Vegetable moussaka
- Grilled veggie wrap
- Make sure to ask for no cheese or yogurt.

MIDDLE EASTERN

- Start with hummus or a spicy muhammara dip, which both make a great dip for veggie grape leaves, or lentil soup.
- Fattoush salad (hold the cheese and pita) or tabbouleh
- Baked falafel or ful mudammas (fava beans) make a hearty side or salad topping.

INDIAN

- Check if the kitchen uses ghee (clarified butter) or vegetable oil. Your orders can often be made without ghee or dairy upon request.

- Start with vegetable samosas or vegetable pakoras.
- Try one of the vegetable dishes, like veggie vindaloo or vegetable curries made with coconut milk.
- Dosa wraps

STEAKHOUSES

- This may seem like a tough spot for a vegan, but steakhouses have the best veggie sides, so create your own vegetable platter.
- Salad with dressing on the side or light on dressing
- French onion soup without cheese
- Any other nondairy soups

DESSERTS

- Sorbets
- Fruit

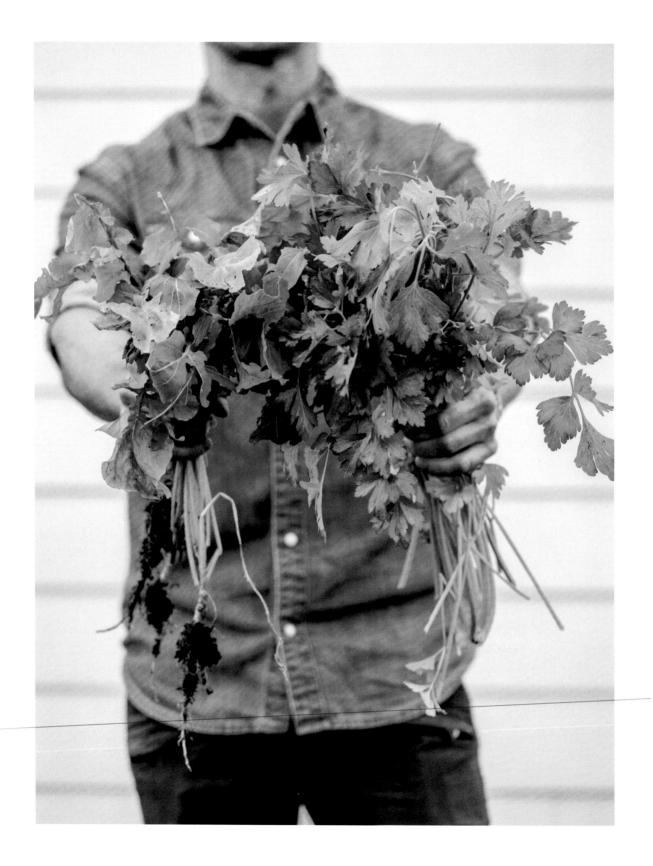

TIPS FOR SUCCESS

BEGINNING ANY NEW HEALTHY lifestyle is an exciting challenge. Try these tips for success to maximize your efforts and results.

1. DRINK WATER

The eight-glasses-per-day rule may be a bit simplistic. The Institute of Medicine suggests that men drink thirteen eight-ounce cups and women drink nine eight-ounce cups a day. Start the day with a glass of water and lemon. This is good for alkalinity, digestion, and rehydration.

Here are a few tips to help you manage fluid intake throughout the day:

- Drink a glass of water/fluid with each meal.
- Drink a glass of water/fluid between each meal.
- Drink a glass of water/fluid before, during, and after exercise.
- Drink more water/fluid when it's hot.
- Don't wait until you're thirsty to drink water; once you are thirsty, you are likely dehydrated.

2. EAT MINDFULLY

This is easy to overlook because most Americans eat while working, reading, or watching TV. Turn off all distractions, focus on your food, and learn to listen to your body's cues. The absolute healthiest way to eat is to 80 percent fullness or just a little bit less than full. So many of us eat until we feel full, and that's simply too much food. This may feel uncomfortable at first if you've become accustomed to that "too full" feeling, but as your body and mind adjust, you'll feel more energized after meals. That's why the plan allows for healthy snacks as needed.

3. EXERCISE FOR AT LEAST 30 MINUTES EACH DAY

Exercise is essential to creating the healthy balance that we all need in order to feel our best. It's important if your goal is to lose weight. Yes, diet counts, and it counts big. Eating plants will reset your body; exercise will make sure the reset sticks.

Diet doesn't excuse you from exercise, and exercise doesn't give you permission to indulge. Successful weight loss is roughly 75 percent diet and 25 percent exercise. There is no amount of exercise that can undo the effects of a poor diet, so exercise for health rather than as an excuse to eat. Once you exercise and feel the positive effects of natural endorphins, you're more likely to embrace healthful foods and have the strength to resist temptation.

4. MAKE TIME FOR YOUR HEALTH

One of the most common hurdles my clients have to overcome while pursuing a healthy lifestyle is finding the time to shop and prepare fresh foods, to eat mindfully, and to exercise. While some of my clients found great success losing weight or getting healthy, others continued to struggle. I began to notice one common behavior consistent with success, and that was the presence of positive habits. Making healthy choices, one seemingly small decision at a time, led to long-term positive results. Start small by replacing one meal a day with a plant-based super plate. Then try eating one meal a day in a quiet, peaceful setting and concentrate on your body's cues. These small steps will add up to a big change.

Be honest with yourself about your habits—especially the ones you want to change. I've found that the people who are most successful at embracing a healthy lifestyle are aware of what their habits were, while unsuccessful people seem unaware that their habits are controlling them. Make a list of what you want to change—take a long walk after dinner, add one plant-based meal per day, eat at the kitchen table instead of on the counter—and take one day at a time.

The choices you make on a daily basis affect your health in the long run. They either get you to the championships, or they keep you on the sidelines. Our habits are the basis for our success—or our failure. If you want to be the best at anything (including the best version of yourself), it all starts with building healthy habits!

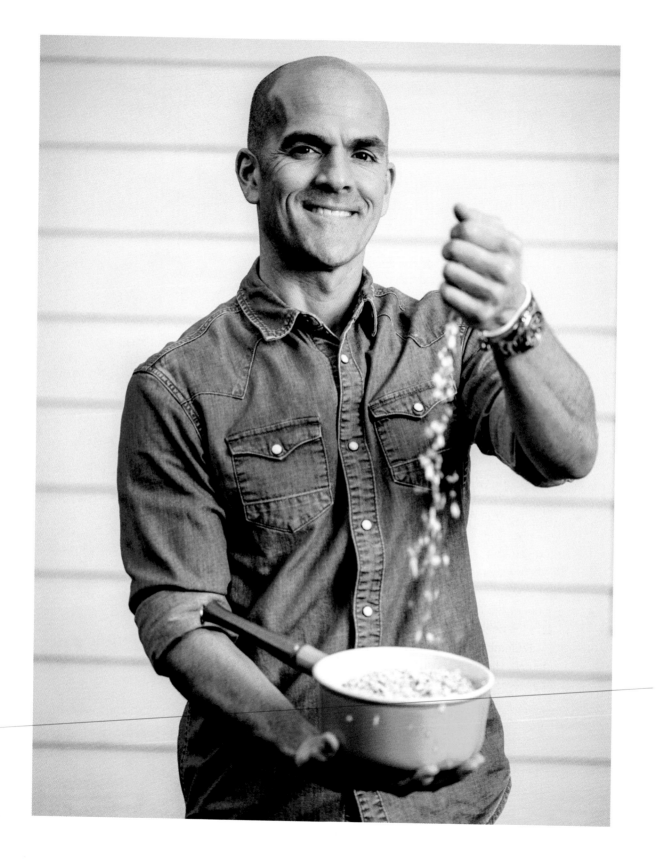

CONCLUSION

ONCE YOU ARE ACCUSTOMED to eating fresh, nutritious food from the earth, dieting is something you'll no longer need to think about. The hard work is changing your habits from unconsciously eating processed food throughout the day to mindfully eating plant-based meals. Once you make delicious, satisfying, healthy plants the staple of your diet, the journey to a healthier lifestyle is easy!

Whether you follow the 22-Day customizable programs outlined in the beginning of the book or begin to incorporate plant-based meals into your life one at a time, you will reap the benefits almost immediately. You have the power to adapt the menus to make the program work for you. Some people remain plant-based eaters for the long haul because they want to continue reaping (or experiencing) the amazing benefits day after day. Some people will just incorporate more vegetables than ever before into their everyday diets. Some people use the challenge as a reset anytime they just want to feel great!

Remember, the goal of any healthy lifestyle change isn't to lose ten pounds again and again—the goal is to create habits that will allow you to lead a balanced life for optimal health. Sustainable results are found by embracing your new healthy habits through deliberate daily practice.

Remember, it takes 21 days to make or break a habit. So as with any lifestyle change, there's a learning curve, a period of discomfort and concerted effort to change your ways. However, the more often you engage in a specific behavior, the more pathways your brain builds to support that behavior, a phenomenon called neuroplasticity. I urge you to fight to build new, healthier habits that will serve you and your family well.

Eating plants is the most powerful, most effective, and simplest way to get healthier. I know because of the incredible impact it has had on the lives of many of my closest friends. My family and I live this life and are fortunate enough to be able to reap the benefits every day. If you want to lose weight, if you want to be fitter and stronger than ever before, you must eat more plants. I've learned firsthand during my twenty years of helping clients lose weight and regain health that diet is the most important tool we have, and that a plant-based diet is the very best way to achieve vitality, longevity, and optimum health—and to get the best body of your life.

This is your time, and this cookbook is the best tool you have to embrace a new, healthier you!

ACKNOWLEDGMENTS

Protect your health. Without it you face a
serious handicap for success and happiness.

—HARRY F. BANKS

I REMAIN FULL OF gratitude and appreciation for the amazing people in my life I have been blessed with.

To my incredibly talented wife, Marilyn, without you, none of these recipes are possible. You make everything more delicious! Thank you for being such a special light in my life. I love you with all my heart!

This project came to life after my dear friend and publisher, Raymond Garcia, believed it was possible and, through his actions, brought an infectious energy to the process that changed everything. Thank you, brother. I love you!

A heartfelt thank-you to my friends and family at Celebra/Penguin Books. Specifically, Jen Schuster, Kim Suarez, Kio Herrera, and Anthony Ramondo.

A special thanks to my friend Sandra Bark for her beautiful abilities and excitement through it all.

Jay and BB, without you, this would not be as fun. I love you both dearly.

A heartfelt thank-you to my mother, Esther, my brother, Alfredo, and my sister, Jennifer, for their constant love and support and to my mother-in-law, Cecilia, for making the most delicious Middle Eastern plant-based meals ever.

A special thanks to our 22-Days family.

Ryan, thank you so much for the wonderful words in this book. You are an inspiring example of how to incorporate a plant-based lifestyle and how to live the life of your dreams. I treasure our friendship and your endless support.

Lastly, a heartfelt thank-you to my best friends, Mila, Maximo, Mateo, Marco Jr., and Marilyn, for their incomparable love and support. You make every day a new gift I will always cherish.

INDEX

WE BELIEVE *in* OURSELVES.

WE BELIEVE THAT

WE BELIEVE THAT SUCCESS IS A BY-PRODUCT OF EFFORT & CONSISTENCY.

WE BELIEVE YOU SHOULD LIVE THE LIFE YOU WANT, NOT JUST *the* ONE YOU HAVE.